FOOD SCIENCE AND TECHNOLOGY

MARINE OILS

(FROM SEA TO PHARMACEUTICALS)

FOOD SCIENCE AND TECHNOLOGY

Additional books in this series can be found on Nova's website
under the Series tab.

Additional e-books in this series can be found on Nova's website
under the e-book tab.

FOOD SCIENCE AND TECHNOLOGY

MARINE OILS

(FROM SEA TO PHARMACEUTICALS)

IOANNIS ZABETAKIS
EDITOR

nova publishers
New York

Library of Congress Cataloging-in-Publication Data

Marine oils : (from sea to pharmaceuticals) / editor Ioannis Zabetakis (Laboratory of Food Chemistry Department of Chemistry, National and Kapodistrian, University of Athens, Greece).
pages cm. -- (Food science and technology)
Includes index.
ISBN 978-1-63463-747-3 (hardcover)
1. Fish oils in human nutrition. 2. Fish oils Health aspects. 3. Drug development. I. Zabetakis, Ioannis.
QP752.F57M37 2015
612.3'97--dc23
2014047182

Published by Nova Science Publishers, Inc. † New York

CONTENTS

PREFACE

In this book, a holistic approach to the concept of fish oils and marine oils has been used in order to evaluate our current knowledge on their availability, biological functions and also their nutritional and commercial value.

We are what we eat. Our food is also what it eats. In other words, if fish are fed better aquafeeds, then we can improve the nutritional value of the final fish product, maximize the added value of the final produce and expand nutraceutical and pharmaceutical applications of fish, fish products and marine oils.

2014 is a historic year. This year is the first year in human history where the amount of fish (as mass in kg) we consume from aquaculture will surpass that from the wild fish. It, thus, becomes quite clear that aquaculture is here to play a vital role in feeding humankind and this role should be performed in a sustainable way. Food security (i.e. producing enough food for all people in a sustainable way) is the top (both political and scientific) priority today and with this book, we try to provoke some thoughts on how we produce fish, how we valorize this fish and what could be done in the future.

For the sustainable production of feeds and food, the biggest challenge is to create sustainable procedures to allow the current and future generations to have unlimited access to food. This challenge is a demanding one: we need to improve our food chain management practices using a more holistic approach in order to lower our high dependency on marine oils (MO). Addressing the aquatic food security, we need to face successfully a "paradox" on the sustainable production of fish feed: today, high amounts of MO are required to produce fish feed. The diminishing levels of available wild fish worldwide combined to the fact that aquacultured carnivorous species require large amounts of wild fish in their feed create an emerging necessity to improve our resource management practices. New, alternative and in a way “non-orthodox” sources of lipids need to be identified and valorized in order to achieve sustainable production of animal and fish feeds and thus increase food security and sustainability.

With the book you are now holding, we are attempting to address the issues of resources management, fish nutritional requirements, aquatic food security, nutritional value of fish and MO and we can exploit MO in the production of nutraceuticals and pharmaceuticals.

In the first chapter, the availability and biochemical value of marine oils (MO) (e.g. composition of MO, various sources and fatty acid composition, krill oils – resources and composition) and their sources are addressed.

In the second chapter, we look into the fish requirements of lipids and how these needs are linked to MO. The compositions of FO/MO and which types of them can be utilized are examined.

In the third chapter, the needs of aquaculture for MO/FO are discussed. We address the issues of sustainability of aquaculture and its dependence on MO.

In the fourth chapter, we discuss the link between MO and diseases. The number one health problem in the world today is CardioVascular Diseases (CVDs) and we discuss how CVDs are linked to the concept of Mediterranean Diet.

In the fifth chapter, we describe the pivotal role that inflammation plays in the development of CVDs and how specific fish/marine components can inhibit inflammation and thus have a cardioprotective role.

In the sixth chapter, we review all the dietary intervention studies (their strengths and their limitations) of fish oils and MO.

In the seventh chapter, the concept of producing pharmaceuticals from MO is presented whilst we have a closer look as to how omega-3 PUFAs are isolated and valorized.

In the eighth chapter, we try to raise questions and food for thought for future nutraceutical and pharmaceutical applications of MO and novel functional foods based on novel functional aquafeeds.

This book would not have been conceived without the constant support and inspiration of two of the most influential teachers of mine, Prof David O’Hagan in St Andrews, Scotland and Prof Constantinos Demopoulos in Athens, Greece.

I had the pleasure to work with David for two years in Durham, England during my post-doc, back in the 90s, and since then David has always helped, in his unique way, to keep my focus. My collaboration with Constantinos started in 1999 when I rang him from Leeds and asked him if he would be interested in some samples of fried cod. The idea was to study the nutritional value of (English) fish and chips and that would be the first of many "fish" papers. From that day, Constantinos has broadened my biochemical horizons so I can now view food as a functional matrix that provides us with flavor as well as cardioprotection.

My most special thanks go to my soulmate and wife, Debbie, not only for reading and commenting on many research papers and the biggest part of this book but for her non-stop encouragement and boundless love. And to Nathaniel and Thiseas, our two boys, for giving me the courage and the optimism to believe that humankind will manage to overcome the growing food insecurity in a fair way for all, especially for the non-privileged.

Dr. Ioannis Zabetakis,
Athens

In: Marine Oils (From Sea to Pharmaceuticals) ISBN: 978-1-63463-747-3
Editor: Ioannis Zabetakis

Chapter 1

SOURCES OF MARINE OILS

Anthony P. Bimbo*
International Fisheries Technology, Kilmarnock, VA, US

ABSTRACT

The demand for marine oil based products continues to evolve and expand. While the main market is for use in aquaculture feeds, primarily for the carnivorous fish, there has been a growing market in the nutraceutical, food and food supplement area as well. The human food market requires the highest levels of omega-3 fatty acids because of label and processing requirements and therefore is willing to pay a premium over what is normally paid by the aquaculture market. There is a finite amount of marine oil produced globally and this volume tends to oscillate periodically when environmental conditions restrict fishing for the primary source, the Peruvian anchoveta. These swings in availability cause swings in the price of these products and that causes availability concerns; will there be sufficient marine oil raw material available for the markets. This chapter will review the evolution of the marine oil market and cover the current and potential future sources of the omega-3 fatty acids which make marine oils desired by both the food and aquaculture segments of the market. Potential future sources include krill, algae, seaweeds, and transgenic plants. Some historical data is presented to preserve the data in a current publication and prevent its loss.

---

* Email apbimbo@verizon.net.

INTRODUCTION

About 71% of the earth's surface is covered by water which is formed into the various oceans, seas, rivers, lakes, and streams. These bodies of water have been very productive over the years, supplying a 10 year average of about 160 million metric tons (mmt) of fish, mollusks, crustaceans, plants, mammals and other creatures from the wild capture and farmed sectors [1]. While fish make up most of the raw material availability (69%), see Figure 1, the wild fish supply from the oceans has reached a flat line so any future supply of fish will have to come from aquaculture if we want to maintain the consumption of fish protein and a supply of the omega-3 fatty acids for food and feed use.

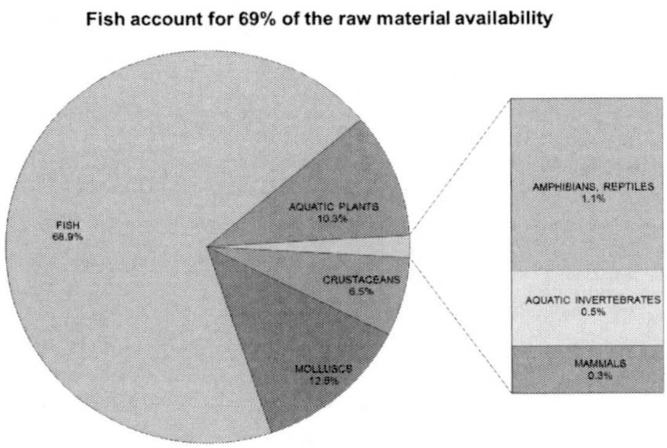

Figure 1. Fish account for 69% of the raw material availability.

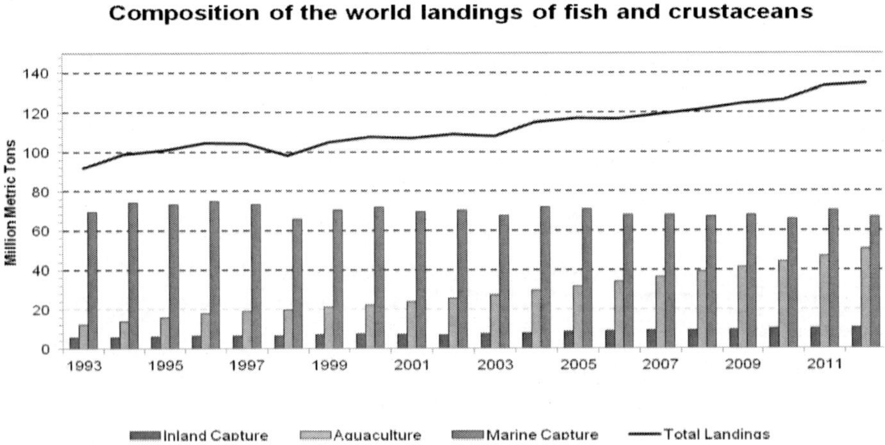

Figure 2. Composition of the world landings of fish and crustaceans.

Figure 2 shows the relative growth in the wild inland and marine capture sectors vs. the growth in combined freshwater and marine aquaculture.

The 10 year average wild fish capture is about 78 and aquaculture production about 33 million metric tons (mmt) or 70% and 30% respectively [1]. Based on the current trends, aquaculture should surpass the wild caught fish volume around the year 2040. This can be seen in Figure 3.

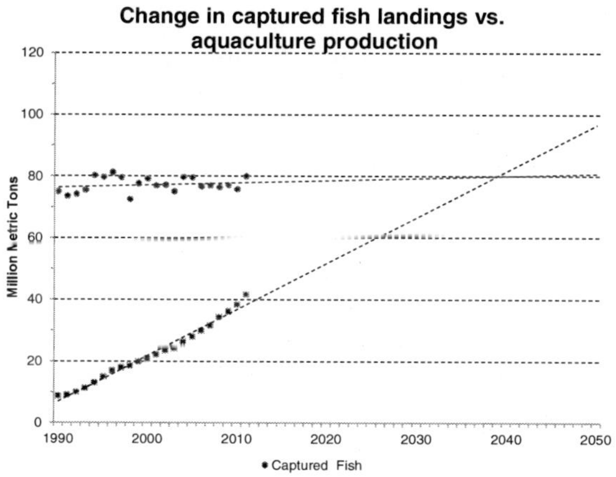

Figure 3. Change in captured fish landings vs. aquacultrure production.

When we look at the disposition of the wild fish catch, which is usually broken down into several end uses, we find that there has been a marked increase in the amount of fish marketed fresh and a drastic decrease in the amount of fish caught specifically for the production of fishmeal and fish oil. However, one must keep in mind that we don't eat the whole fish and depending on the process and product being marketed, the yield loss can range from 40 to 90%. So, while the volume of the targeted species used for fishmeal and oil has been dropping, the waste or by-product from the other markets is also a source or potential source of raw material for fishmeal and oil. In fact about 25-35% of the fishmeal and oil production comes from by-products from the edible fish industry [2,3]. Figure 4 shows how the raw material is utilized in the marketplace, however the product designated for fishmeal and oil use only reflects direct capture for this use and does not include the waste and by-products that can be converted to fishmeal and oil.

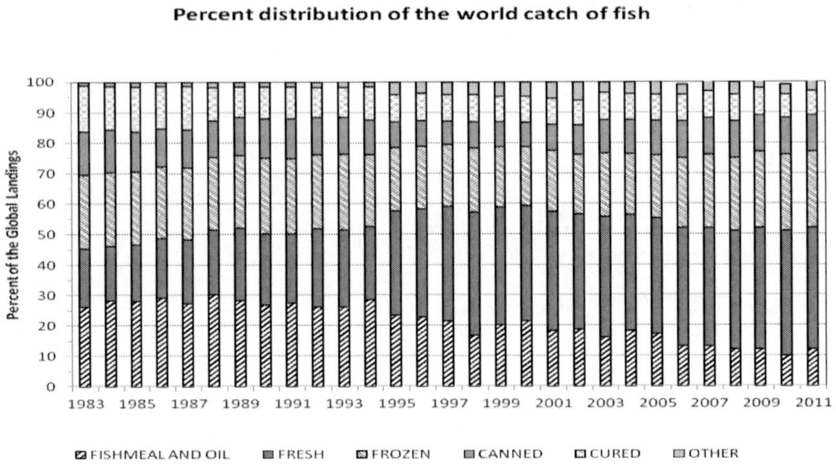

Figure 4. Distribution of the world catch of fish.

Marine Oils in Perspective

Marine oils have been around for a very long time. There are indirect references to them in the Bible [4] and they were consumed during the Roman (27 BC-393 AD) period in fermented fish or Garum [5,6]. Norway was recovering herring oil by primitive pressing during the Viking Period (800 - 1300 AD). By the fourteenth century, cod liver oil was an important by-product for use in lamps and the tanning of leather. Fish oils had been used for centuries for medicinal purposes. Records from the Middle Ages show that cod liver oil was prescribed for rickets. The oil was produced by simply allowing the cod livers to rot. Steam heating of livers to release a better quality oil was introduced about 1850. The identification of vitamin A and D in cod liver oil occurred around 1922 [7].

Prior to 1600 there was relatively little or no demand for oil of any kind. Tallow dips, pine knots, and similar type materials were the principal means of illumination. There was very little machinery in use so lubricants were not needed. The leather industry was undeveloped and the greases used in curing came from the fat of the animal supplying the skin. This was later supplemented by vegetable oils.

Whale oils were used for illumination prior to the seventeenth century, but catching whales in large numbers was not known until around 1870 when the harpoon gun was invented. Prior to that development whale oil was obtained from the few whales that beached on land.

The oil lamp was invented by Aime Argand in 1784 and whale oil became the principal illuminating agent in the early 1800s. It was not only used in residences, but also in street and building lighting. Sperm oil was used in the residences of the wealthy and also in lighthouses, and was the principal illuminant in the coastal lights of the United States, England, Scotland, Ireland, France, and other countries up to 1864. Leather curing increased in importance, and grease for softening was secured in the form of oil from seal, walrus, sea-elephant, and cod livers. As machinery usage increased demand for an enhanced lubricant from sperm oil also increased. Soon other fish oils also became important commercial products, and oils from the livers of cod, haddock, sharks, etc., from herring, menhaden, sardine, pilchard, and other species of the *Clupeidae* family were in general use [7].

There is no global data available pre 1900 but there is data from the US Whaleman's Shipping List covering the period 1860 -1902 for Sperm and Whale oil production [8]. This is shown in Figure 5.

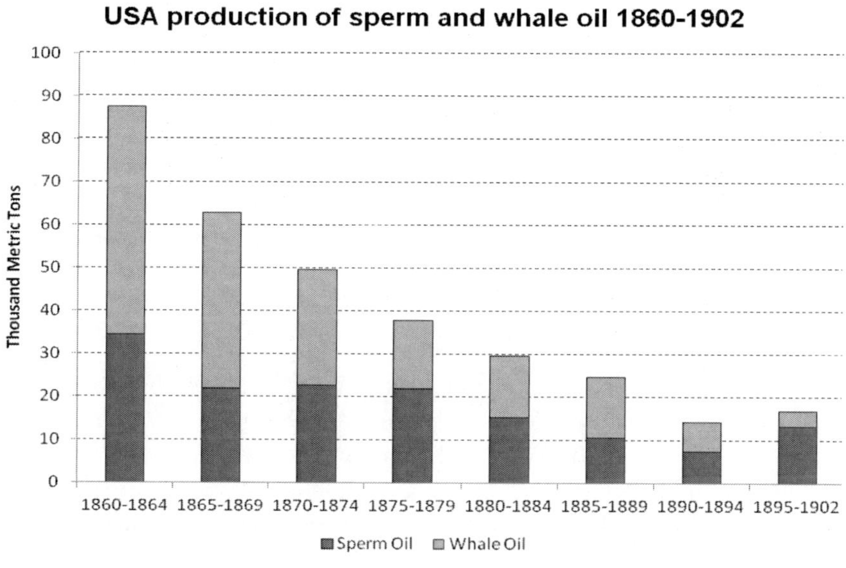

Figure 5. USA production of sperm and whale oil 1860 – 1902.

Historically, global sources of marine oils have evolved over the years. In the period 1938-1955 marine mammal oils (especially from the sperm whale) were the primary source. This changed during the period 1960-1979 when fish body oils displaced the mammal oils. Commercial whaling was prohibited in 1986. Data collected from the FAO statistics and old yearbooks illustrates the changes in the source of production of marine oils over the years [1]. This can be seen in Figure 6.

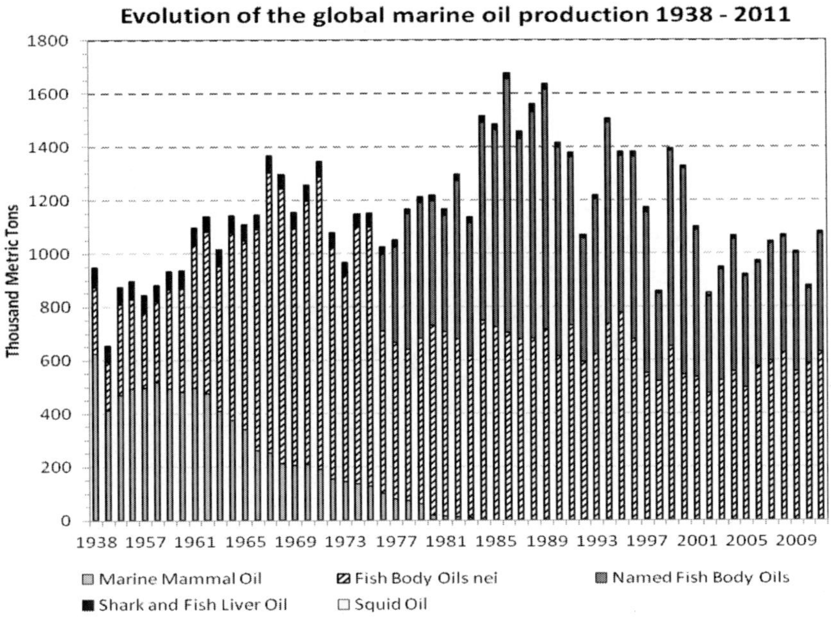

Figure 6. Evolution of the global marine oil production 1938 – 2011.

Unfortunately, the FAO data only identifies the source of about half of the fish oil produced so it is difficult to determine whether the oil is suitable for the omega- 3 market. Half of the oil is simply defined as a fish body oil not easily identified (nie). In some cases the oil probably comes from mixed species so it would be difficult to identify. However, there is no identification of tuna oil within the FAO data even though many countries do identify tuna fishmeal as one of their products. So we are left to wonder, do they produce tuna oil when they produce the fishmeal, is it thrown away, or is it blended with other oils in which case the tuna fishmeal would also be a blend. In some cases, we know that the country produces tuna oil, yet it is not reported. The same would be true for salmon and pollock oil. We know they are produced in the USA and elsewhere, yet they are not listed. The 10 year average production of fish oil appears in Figure 7. Only anchoveta, herring, menhaden, capelin, liver oils, shark and squid oil are mentioned. The krill oil figure is an estimate based on krill landings [1].

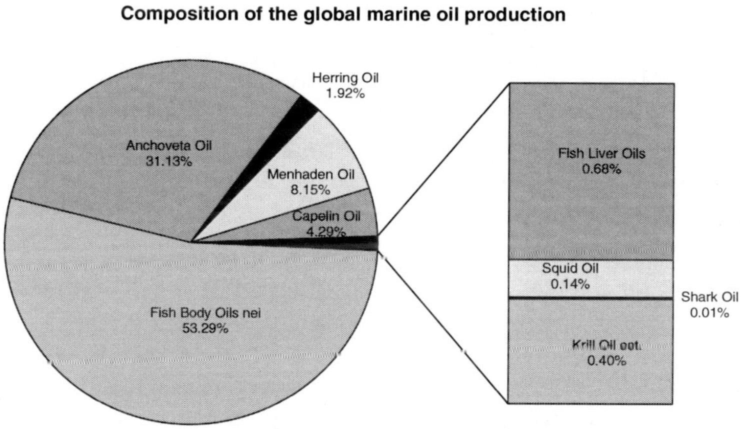

Figure 7. Composition of the global marine oil production [1].

PROCESSING

The raw materials used for the production of marine oils, whether for food use or animal and fish feed come from several sources [9];

- Fish caught specifically for reduction to fishmeal and fish oil such as menhaden, anchovy, capelin, herring and sardines. FAO data indicates that this represents about 19-24 million tons depending on how you define other than food use [1].
- Incidental or by-catch from another fishery, for example the global discards amounted to 27 million metric tons (mmt) with a range of from 18 to 40 mmt with shrimp by-catch accounting for about 11 mmt [10]. A later report estimated that the discards represented about 8% of world's landings (1992-2001) [11]. However a different methodology from that of Alverson et al., was used for this estimate. A more recent report from the UNEP in 2014 mentions that the figure is about 20 million tons annually [12].

- Fish by-products from the edible fisheries (both wild capture and farmed raised) such as cuttings from filleting operations, fish cannery waste, roe fishery waste and more recently surimi processing waste. This group would also include fisheries where there is a mixed use-both for reduction and edible use. This could be about 24 million metric tons.

When we talk about the omega-3 market we could also include krill, squid, seal, single cell organisms, fish roe (eggs) and more recently shrimp/prawn and fishmeal extracts. Genetically modified oilseeds such as soybean, canola/rapeseed and camelina would also fit into the raw material category even though they are not derived from fish.

The original three FAO categories have certain characteristics in common; the fish are of little edible use or the raw material is a waste (left over heads, frames and viscera) and of no edible value and in fact may present a potential disposal problem and the raw material contains a high percentage of oil and or bones [9]. The latter two categories, by-catch and offal produce small volumes of oil compared to the volume produced from whole fish because the traditionally edible species are primarily non-fatty and generally classified as "white fish". However salmon and tuna, for example, do contain oil in the heads and cod, hoki and pollock contain oil in the livers which are processed to provide fish oil.

The processing techniques involved in commercial production of edible fats and oils vary according to the type of raw material. Fish reduction to produce oil and fish meal, except for solvent extraction, generally employs the same principles, techniques and equipment common to the production of the other edible fats and oils. Fish are processed by the wet-reduction method in which the principal operations are cooking, pressing, separation of the oil and water with recovery of oil, and drying of the residual protein material. The separated liquid, after oil removal, is generally evaporated to produce a concentrate which is then added back to the fishmeal during the drying process. Continuous processing from the time the fish are landed optimizes efficiency and maximizes product quality [9]. The wet reduction process is universal and while the equipment might vary and one or two steps omitted, the process is still designed to remove the liquid from the solids, dry the solids and separate the oil from the aqueous liquid (if there is oil). The wet rendering process is used in the majority of the factories that produce fish oil worldwide. Factories all over the world both on land and on ships employ it with slight differences in equipment type. A flow diagram of the wet reduction process is shown in Figure 8.

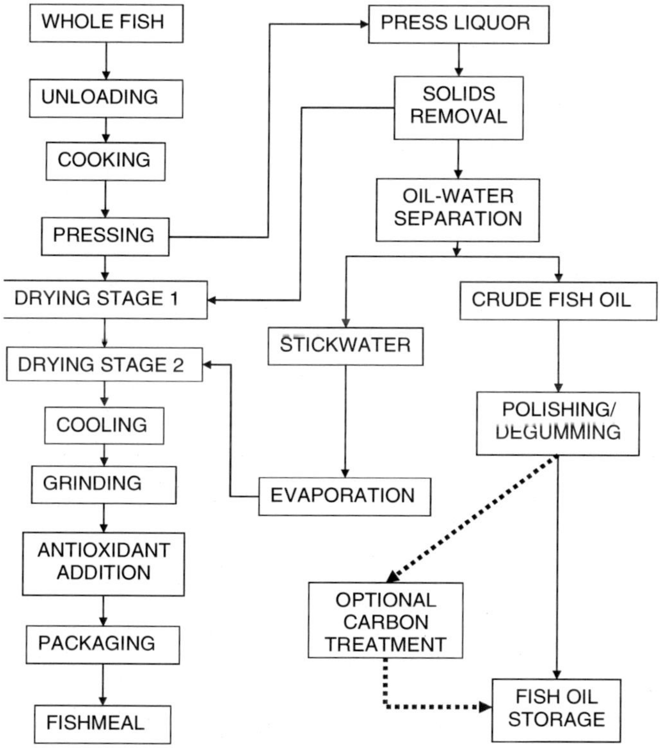

Figure 8. Flow diagram of the wet rendering process [13].

There are a number of other processes that can be used to convert raw fish and cuttings into fish meal and oil.

HYDROLYSIS (ENZYMATIC) AND SILAGE PRODUCTION (AUTOLYTIC)

Hydrolysis involves the use of either external proteolytic enzymes while autolysis involves the use of the natural mix of enzymes contained in the fish viscera. The external enzymes can come from either animal, vegetable or microbial sources and accelerate the breakdown of the proteins into smaller units (peptides). Hydrolysis can also be accomplished chemically by adjusting the pH to either acidic or alkaline conditions. Some of the newer enzymes available today can target peptides with specific lengths and specific functionality [14]. Although the process can be used with any fish, it is primarily used for white fish or offal low in oil. In cases where oily fish are hydrolyzed, the processor must recover the oil phase without denaturing the proteins or face supplying a high fat hydrolyzed protein product or a protein product with reduced functionality. It has been difficult to achieve a commercially viable product from fatty fish that is both functional and low in fat because it usually takes heat to separate the lipid from the aqueous phase and that heat generally will denature the protein.

Silage production is a simplified, low cost, hydrolysis process. It is suited for smaller processing operations because it requires low capital expenses. Fish silage is essentially liquefied fish stabilized against microbial decomposition by an acid. The process involves mincing of the fish followed by the addition of an acid for preservation. The enzymes in the fish gut break down the fish proteins into smaller soluble units and acid helps to speed up their activity while preventing bacterial spoilage. Because the enzyme mix is broad, there is no specificity to peptide chain length or functionality. Acids such as formic, propionic, sulfuric and phosphoric have been used. Generally, the addition of 3-4% acid is sufficient to keep the pH at or below 4.0. If the silage is going to be used in animal feeds the mineral acids should be neutralized before addition to the final product. Silage therefore, might be defined as a crude form of hydrolyzate.

The composition of the silage will be very similar to the starting raw material. Fish silage with the correct pH is stable at room temperature for at least 2 years without decomposition. The protein will continue to hydrolyze and the level of free fatty acids will increase if there is sufficient fish oil present. Silage production offers a solution to the handling of fish waste when the logistics of delivering the waste to a fish reduction plant is not economical. Silage can be produced in large or small containers both on the vessel and on shore. If the silage is processed quickly to recover the oil, it is possible to make an acceptable fish oil product. The silage process can be done in 2 stages, producing a crude silage with very low capital expense and then producing a concentrated silage and fish oil which requires a high capital expense. This two stage process allows production to be done at satellite facilities with the material then transported to a central facility for completion of the processing. Hydrolysis is currently being used to produce krill oil, squid oil and both farmed and wild salmon oil for the omega-3 market.

Dry Rendering

Dry rendering is commonly used to prepare land animal proteins and fats but is not normally used in the manufacture of fish meal and oil. However the process is used with catfish by-products as well as the recent processing of Asian carp in the USA. It is also being used to produce krill meal on vessels in the Antarctic. In this process the raw material is "cooked" to remove the water (essentially the drying process in the fishmeal wet rendering process). The dry oily material is then pressed to remove any oil. Since the water has been removed, the lipid fraction can contain high levels of phospholipids (PLs). In the wet rendering process, the phospholipids hydrate and are recovered with the water fraction. In the dry rendering process, they are not hydrated and therefore remain dissolved in the lipid or oil fraction. Since there is interest in the fish phospholipids, it is possible to produce a PL fraction by hydrating the oil (also called degumming). Further descriptions of this process, which is used in the processing of animal protein by-products has been reviewed [15].

Solvent Extraction

Solvent extraction to produce fish protein concentrate (FPC) is another process that could yield fish oil. Water plus fat constitute about 80% of the whole fish weight, with the fat itself in some species being as high as 20%. The solvent extraction process involves the removal of most of the water and some or all of the fat. Current methods are based mainly on the use of chemical solvents to remove water, fat and fishy tasting components either from the raw fish or from fish meal. The solvents most successfully used in the past were ethanol, hexane, isopropanol, or ethylene dichloride. Normally the solvent is recovered and used over again. The recovered fat is usually part of an azeotropic mixture with water, solvent, and the water soluble components. Separation of this azeotrope to recover the fat sometimes presents problems [16].

In today's omega-3 market, solvent extraction is or can be used to produce krill oil, krill phospholipids, fish phospholipids, fish roe phospholipids, crustacean lipids as well as the single cell oils and transgenic plant oils. For obvious safety reasons solvent extraction cannot be performed on ships where krill are processed.

Super critical Fluid Extraction

This process uses supercritical carbon dioxide as the solvent for removal of highly valuable oils. It has been used to recover lipids from fish roe (eggs) and a commercial process is now in start-up mode to recover the lipid and pigments from shrimp by-products. The capital costs are high but with potential shortages of suitable sources of omega-3 fatty acid oils, companies are turning to these alternative sources and processes. The super critical fluid process has the added benefit of being able to refine and fractionate the oil [17, 18].

Acid-alkali processing

A process that can be used to produce a fish protein isolate and a fish oil by use of alkali and or acid to digest the muscle proteins has been described [19, 20]. Originally developed as a replacement for the surimi process it is now being evaluated as a method for recovery of proteins from fish by-products. If the by-products are from oily fish, then a marine oil product would also be produced..

Raw Materials

The raw materials used for the production of marine oils can come from several sources but generally there are two of them; fish caught specifically for fishmeal and fish oil production (the targeted pelagic fish) and the by-products from the fish caught or farmed for edible purposes. According to FAO data the 5 year average of total landings of fish (wild capture and aquaculture) is 126 mmt for food use and 22 mmt for non-food use or 85% and 15% respectively [1].

Fish Caught Specifically for Fishmeal and Fish Oil Production

It is difficult to pinpoint all of the fisheries specifically destined for the production of fishmeal and oil. In many cases there is an overlap between direct and indirect human consumption markets. According to The Sustainable Fisheries Parnership (SFP), there are 28 fisheries that are targeted specifically for fishmeal and oil production [21]. However SFP tends to separate species by location so herring might appear several times, menhaden twice and sardines and pilchards several times. According to the FAO data the estimated 10 year average volume of fish targeted for fishmeal and oil production is 24 million metric tons (mmt) [1]. These fisheries can be seen in Table 1.

Table 1. Species of fish targeted for the production of fishmeal and oil

Species	Country and % of the catch [1]	10 Year average landings, mmt [1]	Assume 4% fish oil mmt
Peruvian Anchoveta	Peru 77%, Chile 23%	7.29	0.29
Other Anchovy sp.	China 30%, Turkey 9%, Thailand 5%, Japan 14%, South Korea 9%, Mexico 3%, South Africa 8%, Indonesia 2%, Philippines 3%, India 3%, Ghana 2%, Italy 2%, Panama 2%, Others 4%	2.66	0.11
Sandeels	China 36%, Denmark 53%, Norway 11%	0.45	0.02
Herring	Norway 30%, Iceland 10%, Russian Federation 14%, Denmark 4%, Finland 3%, Canada 6%, UK 3%, USA 4%, Netherlands 3%, Sweden 3%, Faeroe Islands 3%, Germany 2%, Mexico 5%, Japan 2%	2.63	0.11
Atlantic and Gulf Menhaden	USA 100%	0.675	0.03
Sprat	Denmark 38%, Sweden 17%, Poland 13%,Latvia 10%, Estonia 8%, Russian Federation 5%, Iran 4%, Chile 7%	0.51	0.02
Pilchard	Morocco 35%, Mexico 27%, Portugal 4%, Algeria 3%, USA 2%, Croatia 1%, Spain, 2%, Turkey 1%, Netherlands 2%, Japan 4%, China 8%, South Africa 10%, Namibia 1%	1.8	0.07
Araucanian Herring (Chilean Sardine)	Chile 100%	0.58	0.02

Table 1. (Continued)

Species	Country and % of the catch[1]	10 Year average landings, mmt [1]	Assume 4% fish oil mmt
Sardinella sp.	Philippines 25%, Indonesia 19%, Senegal 17%, Morocco 5%, Venezuela/Bolivia 6%, Mauritania 5%, Nigeria 5%, Angola 5%, Thailand 6%, Belize 3%, Brazil 5%	1.4	0.06
Indian Oil Sardine	India 77%, Yemen 9%, Oman 9%, Iran 6%	0.4	0.02
Chilean Jack Mackerel	Chile 74%, China 8%, Peru 13%, Vanuatu 5%	1.3	0.05
Other Horse Mackerels	China 5%, Indonesia 4%, Namibia 16%, Japan 11%, Belize 7%, India 7%, Mauritania 3%, Lithuania 3%, New Zealand 3%, Philippines 4%, Spain 3%, Thailand 3%, Netherlands 5% , Others 26%.	1.6	0.06
Capelin	Iceland 54%, Norway 25%,Canada 5%, Faeroe Islands 3%, Greenland 2%, Russian Federation 6%, Others 5%	0.64	0.03
Norway Pout	Denmark 61%, Norway 37%, Faeroe Islands 2%	0.04	0.002
Pacific Thread Herring	Mexico 68%, Panama 15%, Ecuador 9%, Venezuela 3%, Brazil 4%	0.21	0.06
Blue Whiting and Southern Blue Whiting	Norway 32%, Russian Federation 16%, Iceland 15% Faeroe Islands 13%, Netherlands 4%, UK 3%, New Zealand 2%, Chile 2%, Argentina 2%, Ireland 2%, Spain 2%, Others 7%	1.45	0.01005
Boarfish	Ireland 73%, Denmark 23%, UK 5%	0.038	0.002
Totals		23.67	0.96

Most of this catch is concentrated in 13 fisheries as shown in Table 1. Asuming a conservative fish oil yield of 4%, they also represent about 96% of the world fish oil production of about 1 million metric tons.

By-products from Wild Caught Fish Converted to Fish Oil Production

The FAO data does not report how much fish by-product material is produced and converted to fishmeal and oil. FAO only reports how much fish is captured for industrial applications and that was shown in Table 1. While the yield of edible meat from fish varies by the species and the end use of the fish, a general assumption that 46% of the fish is waste or by-product will be used in this chapter. For example, not all the edible fish are landed in edible condition so they may be discarded and used for industrial purposes. Some edible fish are processed at sea and the waste may or may not be further processed into fishmeal and oil. Fish may be discarded overboard simply because they are too small or would impact the fishing vessel's quota for that species. So, while 46% may be a good figure for the amount of by-product that could be generated from the fish, it would only be the theoretical estimate of what could be available and not what is actually collected. For, conservative calculations we could also assume that 50% of the available waste is actually collected and converted into fishmeal and oil. Table 2 shows some of the species' by-products known to be used for fishmeal and oil production.

Table 2. Species of fish targeted primarily for edible purposes with the waste potentially designated for fishmeal and oil production

Species	Country and % [1]	10 Year Average Landings, mmt [1]	Assume 46% Waste mmt	Assume 50% Waste Recovered mmt	Assume 3% Fish Oil mmt
Shad	Bangladesh 67%, Sierra Leone 16%, Guinea 9%, Cameroon 9%	0.43	0.2	0.1	0.003
Tuna and Bonito sp.	Indonesia 15%, Philippines 10%, Japan 9%, Taiwan 7%, Ecuador 4%, South Korea 5%, Spain 5%, USA 3%, Papua New Guinea 4%, Iran 3%, China 3%, Mexico 2%, Sri Lanka 2%, India 2%, Maldives 2%, France 2%, Panama 2%, Others 20%	5.6	2.58	1.29	0.0387

Table 2. (Continued)

Species	Country and % [1]	10 Year Average Landings, mmt [1]	Assume 46% Waste mmt	Assume 50% Waste Recovered mmt	Assume 3% Fish Oil mmt
Mackerel sp.	China 12%, Chile 7%, Indonesia 11%, Japan 13%, Thailand 5%, Malaysia 4%, Norway 4%, U K 4%, South Korea 4%, Iceland 2%, Philippines 4%, India 3%, Morocco 2%, Russian Federation 2%, Taiwan 2%, Peru 2%, Others 19%.	3.82	1.76	0.88	0.026
Alaska Pollock	Russian Federation 44%, USA 45%, Japan 8%, Others 3%	2.86	1.32	0.66	0.0198
Atlantic Cod	Norway 28%, Russian Federation 26%, Iceland 21%, Denmark 3%, Faeroe Islands 4%, UK 2%, Germany 2%, Poland 2%, Canada 2%, Others 10%	0.9	0.41	0.205	0.00615
Pacific Cod	USA 68%, Russian Federation 17%, Japan 12%, South Korea 2%	0.39	0.18	0.09	0.0027
Wild Salmon and Trout	USA 31%, Russian Federation 32%, Japan 34%, Canada 2%	1.1	0.51	0.255	0.00765
Hake sp.	Argentina 28%, Canada 6%, Chile 11%, Namibia 19%, Peru 2%, USA 13%, Uruguay 2%, Others 19%	1.37	0.63	0.315	0.00945
Blue Grenadier (Hoki)	New Zealand 88%, Others 12%	0.14	0.06	0.03	0.0009
Pacific Saury	Japan 55%, Taiwan 24%, Russian Federation 15%	0.47	0.22	0.11	0.003
Totals		17.08	7.87	3.94	0.12

BY-PRODUCTS FROM FARMED FISH CONVERTED TO FISH OIL PRODUCTION

In addition to the wild fish destined for the food market, there is a considerable amount of farmed fish produced. Farmed fish production is increasing at a rapid rate and is expected to reach the wild caught fish production by the year 2040 [22]. As with the wild fish, the waste could be about 46% of the live weight thus presenting us with an additional amount of potential raw material available for the omega-3 or marine oil market. Table 3 shows some of the major farmed fish raised for food use and an estimate of how much waste and fish oil might be produced from the waste.

Table 3. Species of farmed fish targeted or potentially targeted for food use and the by-products converted or can be converted to fishmeal and oil production

Species	Country and %	10 Year Average Landings, mmt [1]	Assume 46% Waste mmt	Assume 50% Waste Recovered mmt	Assume 3% Fish Oil mmt
Farmed Salmon and Trout	Canada 4%, Chile 25%, Faeroe Islands 2%,Iran 3%, Norway 37%, Turkey 3%, U K 6%, Others 19%	2.3	1.06	0.53	0.0159
Chinese Farmed Freshwater Fish	China 100%	18.41	8.47	4.235	0.12705
Chinese Farmed Marine Fish	China 100%	0.69	0.32	0.16	0.0048
Farmed Channel Catfish	USA 58%, China 40%, Others 2%	0.4	0.18	0.09	0.0027
Farmed Pangas Catfish	Vietnam 85%, Indonesia 12%, Others 3%	0.94	0.43	0.215	0.00645
Other Farmed Catfish	China 28%, Indonesia 15%, Bangladesh 14%, Nigeria 6%, Others 37%	1.6	0.74	0.37	0.0111
Farmed eels	China 71%, Denmark (1%), Indonesia (1%), Japan 9%, S. Korea (2%), Netherlands 2%, Taiwan 12%, Italy 1, Malaysia 1%	0.24	0.11	0.06	0.0017
Totals		24.58	11.31	5.66	0.17

Shellfish Currently Converted to Fish Oil Production or By-products That Could Be Converted to Fish Oil Production

Shellfish include mollusks and crustaceans. Squid is a mollusk, krill, shrimp and prawns are crustaceans and all are used in the production of meals or hydrolyzates and oils. Krill and squid oils are routinely used in the omega-3 market. Generally shrimp and prawn waste is dried and sold as a shellfish meal for animal feed diets. One estimate is that 60% of the crustacean landings are waste. Recently, a group in Canada announced the startup of a company that will extract the lipid and pigments from shrimp waste with supercritical carbon dioxide. This oil will be used in the omega-3 market. If that use works then there is potentially a very large resource of raw material for this market. Table 4 lists some of the shellfish species that are used or might be used in the future for omega-3 production.

Table 4. Species of shellfish designated for edible or industrial use with the waste from the edilbe species a potential source of omega-3 oil

	Country and %	10 Year Average Landings, mmt	Assume 46% Waste mmt	Assume 50% Waste Recovered mmt	Assume 3% Fish Oil mmt
Squid [1]	China 24%, Peru 14%, Japan 9%, South Korea 10%, Argentina 5%, Taiwan 4%, Indonesia 2%, Thailand 2%, Philippines 2%, USA 3%, Falkland Is. 2%, Malaysia 2%, New Zealand 2%, Chile 6%, Others 12%	2.34	1.08	0.54	0.016
Farmed Shrimp and Prawns [1]	China 49%, Ecuador 3%,India 3%, Indonesia 7%,Mexico 2%, Thailand 10%, Vietnam 8%, Others 17%	4.79	2.2	1.1	0.033
Wild Shrimp and Prawns [1]	China 37%, India 12%, Indonesia 7%, Vietnam 4%, Canada 5%, USA 4%, Malaysia 3%, Greenland 4%, Mexico 2%, Thailand	3.2	1.47	0.735	0.022

	Country and %	10 Year Average Landings, mmt	Assume 46% Waste mmt	Assume 50% Waste Recovered mmt	Assume 3% Fish Oil mmt
	2%, Others 20%				
Antarctic Krill [23]	Norway 33%, South Korea 23%, China 2%, India 2%,Japan 21%,Poland 5%, Ukraine 5%, Vanuatu 5%, Others 4%	0.15	0.15[1]	0.15	0.005
Totals		10.48	4.90	2.53	0.08

[1] Assume all the krill is used for krill meal and oil production and the oil yield is 3%.

The by-products and waste from the edible fisheries (both wild capture and aquaculture), therefore represent alternative sources of products for the marine oil markets.

The difficulty in pinpointing or matching fisheries with fish oil production is complex. The major source of data for fisheries production is the FAO statistical databases [1]. The data is generally about 2 years behind since it takes that long to collect the information from the many developed and developing countries. FAO also reports commodity information and that is usually 3 years behind. Unfortunately, FAO does not report the commodities by species, so most of the data is generic fish oil not easily identified (nei). On the other hand, the statistical publication Oil World is generally up to date and reports production, imports, exports and consumption of most of the commodity products including fish oil. But Oil World is commodity oriented and does not identify the species from which the oil comes, it only reports fish oil production and country of origin. It is possible that Oil World cannot get the information from many of the smaller producers so there is a relatively large 'others' category. This 'others' category contains some of the producers of tuna and krill oil, for example. So, what is needed is a bridge between the two data sources. Considering the need for this information from the growing omega-3 market, it would seem to be an important goal and perhaps as the market grows and demand for this information increases, we might see it in the future.

Fish Oil

Introduction

Presently 7 entities represent most of the global marine oil production. This can be seen in Figure 9.

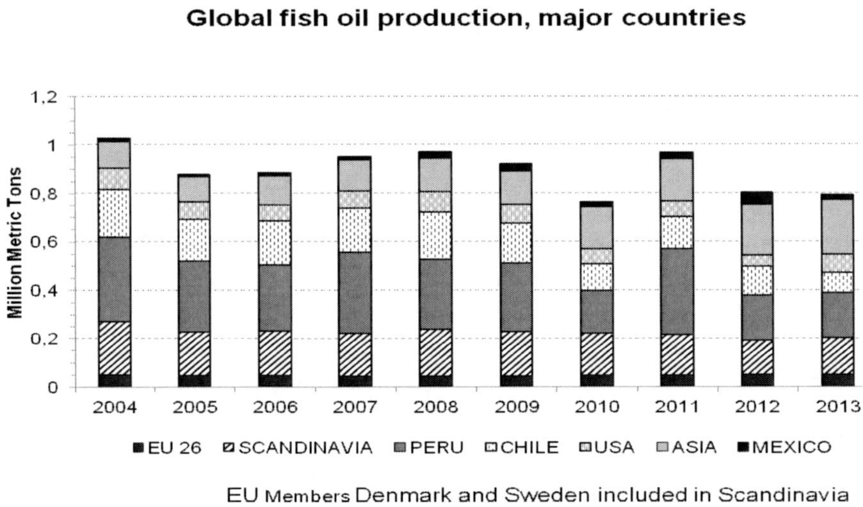

Figure 9. Global fish oil production, major countries [24].

While these 7 entities represent approximately 90% of the production, there are a number of countries included in the other 10% of the production. Some of these are shown in Figure 10. Even with these additional countries, there is still an additional group of 'others' representing about 25,000 tons of fish oil which could be of great interest to the omega-3 producers in different regions in the future.

The market for fish oil has been evolving for a long time. Originally used as an industrial oil for illumination, tanning leather and in coatings and paints it moved to food use when hydrogenation for the production of shortenings and margarine became available. It then moved to farmed fish feeds, pet foods and now the omega-3 market. In almost every case the price has also evolved and the succeeding market was willing to pay a premium over what the existing market was paying. Currently we are in the midst of a similar situation with competition between the farmed fish and omega-3 markets.

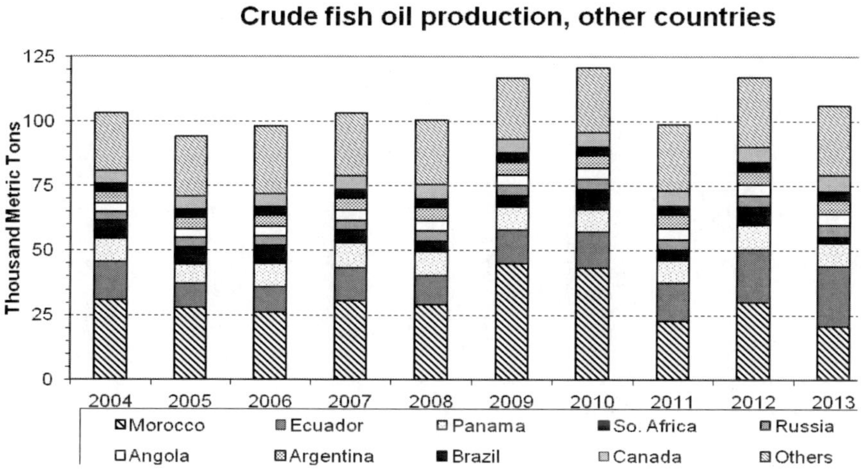

Figure 10. Global fish oil production, other countries [24].

The evolution of the marine oil market by end use is shown in Figure 11. There has been a displacement of the hydrogenation market by the aquaculture market over most of this period. However, the Omega-3 market is beginning to displace some of the other uses and will eventually begin to pressure the aquaculture market.

The omega-3 market is composed of natural triglyceride oils as well as concentrated fatty acids, ethyl esters and re-esterified triglycerides. During the production of these concentrates yields are reduced as the non-omega-3 fractions are removed along with glycerine and some omega-3s. As the relative volume of concentrate production increases compared to the natural triglyceride oils there will be an increasing demand on the raw material sources and this will eventually require new sources of these fatty acids. There will also be continuing pressure on the producers to investigate newer technologies that recover more of the omega-3 fatty acids in the raw material. As the relative concentrate volume increases, more demand for efficiency will be essential as the price of the raw materials will also increase. The difference between raw material and finished product (yield) is shown in Figure 12.

It is difficult to project the overall demand for crude fish oil to supply these markets since not all fish oil is presently suitable. Most of the market is pursuing anchovy and sardine oils, which puts a heavy strain on that supply. This is another reason to find alternative, suitable sources of omega-3 oils.

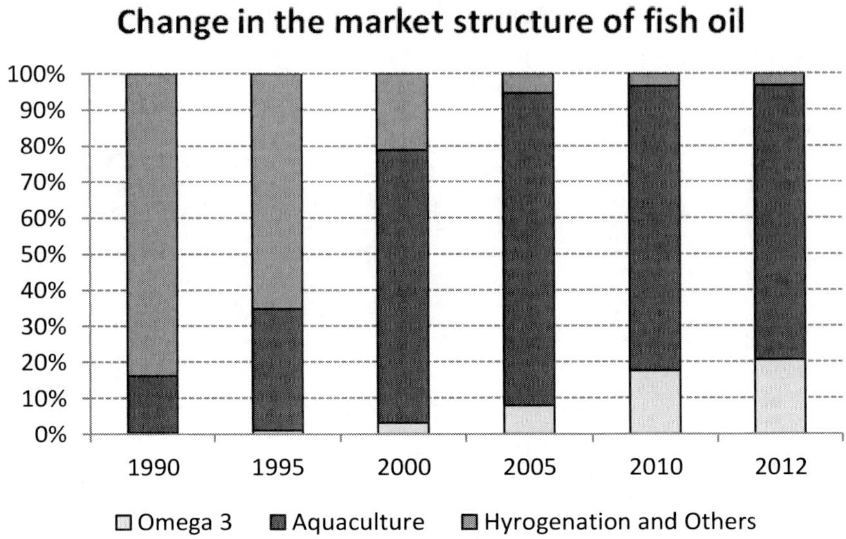

Figure 11. Change in the market structure for fish oil [25, 26].

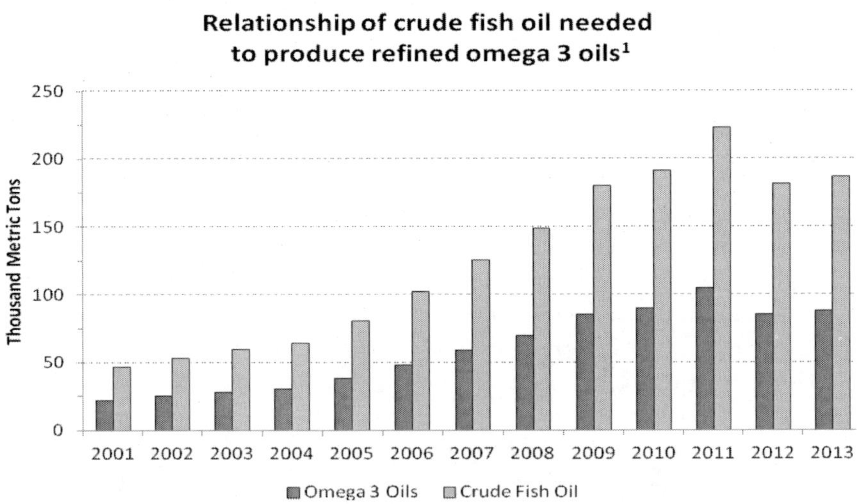

[1] Based on a product mix of 90% triglyceride oils and 10% concentrates.

Figure 12. Relationship of crude fish oil needed to produce refined omega-3 oils [27, 28].

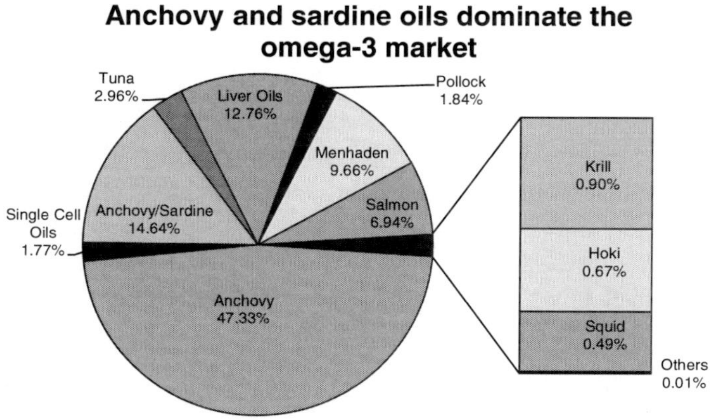

Figure 13. Anchovy and sardine oils dominate the omega-3 market [28].

Anchovy and sardine oils account for about 62% of the raw materials for the omega-3 market. Because of their composition, these oils form the base for the market with other oils from krill, menhaden, salmon, cod and tuna meeting niche global markets. This can be seen in Figure 13.

MARINE OIL COMPOSITION

While anchovy and sardine oils dominate the omega-3 market, all marine oils have a place in this market. The main consideration is first of all how much total omega-3 is in the oil and can you recover it through some method of separation that is economically feasible. In the past, oils such as capelin, herring, salmon, and pollock were considered marginal at best because they did not have the optimum levels of eicosapentaenoic acid (EPA) and docosahexaenoic acid (DHA) or total omega-3 fatty acids (30-35%). But with the market moving away from natural oils and towards concentrates, the source seems less important than the economics to recover the omega-3s in the oil. So today, we see products produced from wild and farmed salmon, pollock, herring and even oil extracted from shrimp waste and phospholipids extracted from fishmeal. One concept that was considered impossible some years ago, the sale of virgin or crude oils for human consumption is now mainstream and sells into the natural food markets. Therefore, knowing the composition of the raw materials becomes a critical part of the success in penetrating this market.

There have been many papers published on the composition of the lipid in various species of whole fish; both the edible portions and waste. From the perspective of consuming the edible flesh, a simple extraction of the lipid in the flesh is suitable for determining the omega-3 content in the flesh. The difficulty with this procedure with by-products and waste is that you generally want to recover the oil in the waste and extracting it with a solvent or the Bligh and Dyer Method (B&D) [29] for total lipid extracts does not necessarily reflect what you would get if you rendered the waste. While krill, phospholipids in fishmeal and krill meal are extracted with a solvent, in most other cases the waste is steam cooked and the oil recovered from the liquors by pressing and liquid separation. You may not get the same type of oil in rendering that you would get when you use the B&D Method. The B&D method will extract the phospholipids which are generally high in EPA and or DHA, while the neutral oil that is recovered by rendering may not have as much of these fatty acids. The wet rendering process essentially removes the phospholipid fraction with the water phase. This water phase is evaporated and added back to the fishmeal. So the recovered oil in the wet rendering process is mostly triglyceride with some fatty acids and a small amount of phospholipids. I have been suggesting that researchers simply take the waste or fish parts and put them into a boil in a bag type container and cook them, then recover the oil and analyze it for the omega-3 content. This would go a long way in determining what is and isn't suitable for the omega-3 market. Dry rendering, on the other hand removes the water first so the phospholipids dissolve in the oil and are recovered with the oil fraction. Unfortunately only a few plants use the dry rendering process to produce fish oil.

Fish Fatty Acid Composition

Table 5 compares the levels of fatty acids in the lipid of the various current and potential alternative sources of oil for the omega-3 market. Where the composition represents oil, this is noted. In all other cases the lipid represents a solvent extract predominantly by the B&D method.

Table 5. Omega-3 fatty acid content of oil from fish targeted for fish oil production

	% Total fatty acids								
Species	Saturates	Mono-unsaturates	C18:2 n-6	C18:3 n-3	C20:5 n-3	C22:5 n-3	C22:6 n-3	EPA+ DHA	Total omega-3
Peruvian anchovy oil [30, 31]	31	25	1	3	20	2	9	29	35
Peruvian anchovy oil [43]	32	23	1	1	20	2	14	34	39
Aracunha herring (Chilean sardine) oil [32, 33]	35	24	3	2	15	3	10	25	32
Indian oil sardine [34, 35, 36]	39	22	2	2	15	2	14	29	36
Bali sardinella [37]	47	29			3		14	17	
Japanese sardine oil [38, 39 40,]	30	29	1	3	15	2	8	23	30
Atlantic/North Sea herring oil [31,38]	25	52	2	4	6	1	7	13	20
Herring oil [43]	24	46	1	1	7	1	10	17	21
Thread herring [41]	42	20	1	1	6	2	19	25	29
Sprat oil [30]	26	47	2		6	1	9	15	18
Sprat oil [43]	23	45	1	1	6	1	10	16	21
Atlantic menhaden oil [42]	32	22	1	3	13	2	10	23	32
Atlantic menhaden stearine [43]	47	19	1	1	12	2	8	20	30
Gulf menhaden oil [42]	31	25	1	2	13	2	7	20	27
Menhaden oil [43]	36	25	1	1	13	2	8	21	27
Chilean jack mackerel oil [33, 44, 45]	29	30	1	2	11	2	16	27	31
Norway pout oil [30, 46, 47]	21	36	1	2	11	1	20	31	35
Blue whiting oil [47, 48]	23	25	1	3	12	1	26	38	43
Capelin oil [30, 49,50]	19	57	1	1	9	1	6	15	17
Sand eel oil [30, 49, 50]	24	40	1	5	12	1	12	24	31
Japanese anchovy oil [43]	27	32	2	1	12	1	12	24	33
Pacific saury oil [43]	20	45	1	1	7	1	10	17	27
California sardine oil [43]	38	22	1	1	14	1	17	32	33
Boarfish oil [43]	23	50	1	1	4	2	10	14	18

Table 6. Omega-3 fatty acid content of oil and lipids from edible fish with the by-product converted to fish oil

	% Total fatty acids								
Species	Saturates	Mono-unsaturates	C18:2 n-6	C18:3 n-3	C20:5 n-3	C22:5 n-3	C22:6 n-3	EPA+ DHA	Total omega-3
European anchovy [51,52,53, 54]	33	25	2	1	9	1	16	25	28
Black Sea anchovy [53]	36	29	3	1	10	1	16	26	30
Brazil enchova [55]	33	37	3		4	2	13	17	23
Northern anchovy [56]	41	20	1		16	3	16	32	35
Northern anchovy oil [43, 56]	27	28	1	1	20	2	9	29	36
Spanish sardine [41]	38	17	1	1	6	1	27	33	36
Pacific sardine [56]	41	21	1		19	4	10	29	34
Brazil sardine [55]	40	20	2		9	1	23	32	35
So. African pilchard oil [31]	30	24	1	2	19	2	6	25	34
Portuguese sardine oil [31]	31	28	1	3	11	1	13	24	32
Pacific herring [57]	28	48		1	9	1	9	18	21
Atlantic horse mackerel [58]	24	34	1	1	5	1	10	15	18
Japanese horse mackerel [59]	25	23	4	4	7	2	13	20	23
Blue whiting [47,48, 62]	23	25	1	3	12	1	26	38	43
Blue whiting oil [30]	21	48	2	1	7	1	11	18	22
Indian mackerel [36]	36	22	2	2	10	2	17	27	32
Spanish mackerel [36]	47	26	1	1	5	1	14	27	22
Spotted mackerel [61]	36	22		1	6	2	18	24	27
Atlantic mackerel [62]	30	30	2		8	1	12	20	22
Atlantic mackerel oil [43]	21	30	2	1	6	1	11	17	27
Chub mackerel [63]	35	23	1	1	5	3	21	26	30
Chub mackerel oil [43]	25	37	2	1	9	2	12	21	30

	% Total fatty acids								
Species	Saturates	Mono-unsaturates	C18:2 n-6	C18:3 n-3	C20:5 n-3	C22:5 n-3	C22:6 n-3	EPA+ DHA	Total omega-3
Mediterranean horse mackerel [64]	36	16			6	1	35	41	44
Black Sea horse mackerel [65, 66]	38	31				1	17	19	21
Cod liver, Atlantic[43]	18	43	3	3	11	1	13	24	31
Cod liver, Pacific [43]	9	54	1	1	10	3	13	20	30
Cod liver oil Spain [67]	21	43	1	2	9	1	11	20	25
Cod liver oil Sweden [68]	21	44	2	3	10	1	15	25	27
Cod liver oil Poland [68]	19	52		2	9	1	12	21	23
Cod liver oil Poland [68]	23	44	1	2	10	3	13	23	26
Cod liver oil Iceland [68]	18	53	1	2	10	1	13	23	24
Cod Liver oil [43]	17	52	2	1	9	1	12	21	27
Wild Pacific salmon oil [70, 43]	20	33	1	2	8	3	10	18	25
Wild Atlantic salmon [71,72]	25	43	2	1	6	2	9	15	19
Alaska pollock liver oil [30,73,74]	21	47		2	10	1	5	15	18
Pollock oil [43]	18	57	1	1	10	1	5	15	19
Blue Grenadier (hoki) [75, 76]	31	23			6	2	35	41	43
Argentine hake [77]	22	40		4	7		14	21	29
Yellow fin tuna [36]	35	19	1	3	7	2	21	28	33
Albacore tuna [48]	32	29			6	1	26	32	33
Skipjack tuna [48]	33	32			8	2	20	28	30
Tuna oil nei [30, 48, 68, 78, 79,80,81, 82]	30	27	1	1	8	2	23	31	36
Tuna oil [43]	31	26	1	1	6	1	27	33	37

Table 6. (Continued)

	% Total fatty acids								
Species	Saturates	Mono-unsaturates	C18:2 n-6	C18:3 n-3	C20:5 n-3	C22:5 n-3	C22:6 n-3	EPA+ DHA	Total omega-3
Farmed Atlantic salmon oil, Chile [83]	26	34	3	1	10	5	14	24	32
Farmed salmon, Turkey [54]	28	35	11	1	3	2	17	20	24
Farmed Atlantic salmon [82]	24	31	7		7	4	16	23	27
Farmed salmon oil [43]	19	54	21	7	5	2	6	11	21
Farmed Atlantic salmon, Tasmania [84]	30	33	2		8	3	20	28	32
Farmed king salmon oil New Zealand [85]	17	21	4		4	1	6	10	12
Farmed channel catfish USA [86, 87, 88]	25	51	13	1	1	1	3	4	6
Farmed catfish, Japan [86]	27	28	4	1	3	2	18	21	24
Tra catfish [84]	43	35	8	1		1	5	5	7
Freshwater eel [89]	27	56	5				3	3	5
Freshwater swamp eel (China) [101]	28	35	14	4	2	1	5	7	12
Marine Pike eel (China)	36	34	1	1	5	2	14	19	22
Short Fin Eel, wild [146]	31	42	1	1	4	3	7	11	16
Short fin eel, farmed1 [146]	30	41	4	1	7	4	6	13	20
Short Fin eel, farmed2 [146]	29	39	3	1	6	4	11	17	24

Table 7. Omega-3 fatty acid content of krill lipids, krill fractions and krill oil products

	% Total fatty acids								
Species	Saturates	Monoenes	C18:3 n-3	C18:4 n-3	C20:5 n-3	C22:5 n-3	C22:6 n-3	EPA+DHA	Total omega-3
Whole krill oil [91]	24	19	1		15	1	6	21	24
Whole krill oil [92]	35	28		4	17	1	10	27	31
Whole krill lipid [93]	37	30	1	3	15	1	8	23	28
Krill oil [43]	27	17	2	4	20		11	31	38
Phospholipid fraction [93]	18	20			23	1	33	56	58
Triglyceride fraction [93]	46	38	1	3	4		1	5	10
Whole krill *E.superba* [94]	37	31	1	3	13		8	21	26
Whole krill nei [94]	27	27	1	1	13	1	18	31	36
E. superba total lipid [94]	29	18	2	4	25		15	40	48
E superba phosphatidyl choline [94]	30	17	2	5	23		12	35	43
E. superba phosphatidyl ethanolamine [94]	23	23	1	1	20		21	41	43
E. superba lyso phosphatidyl choline [94]	45	17		1	7		3	10	13
E. crystallorophias total lipid [94]	33	27	1	2	19		9	28	31
E. crystallorophias phosphatidyl choline [94]	35	28	2	2	15		5	20	24
E. crystallorophias phosphatidyl ethanolamine [94]	34	33			15		10	25	26
E. crystallorophias lyso phosphatidyl choline [94]	41	16			2			2	2

Table 8. Omega-3 fatty acid content of oils and lipids from various squid

	% Total fatty acids								
Species	Saturates	Mono-unsaturates	C18:3 n-3	C18:4 n-3	C20:5 n-3	C22:5 n-3	C22:6 n-3	EPA+ DHA	Total omega-3
Squid nei [39,46, 76, 95]	30	28		2	10	1	27	37	42
Arrow Squid [48]	31	20			14	1	38	52	52
Flying Squid [47]	26	8			18		44	62	
Magister Armhook Squid medium [50]	22	35	1	1	13		20	33	37
North Pacific Bobtail Squid [50]	23	29			19	1	20	39	41
Indian squid [96]	41	14	2		8		12	20	27
Broad Squid [48]	35	14			14	1	34	48	49
Squid nei mantle lipids [96]	34	10			15		37	52	52
Squid nei liver lipids [96]	23	39	1	1	11	1	15	26	30
Squids, nei [96]	33	18	1		15	2	28	43	46

Table 9. Omega-3 fatty acid content of shrimp, prawns and other shellfish

	% Total fatty acids								
Species	Saturates	Mono-unsaturates	C18:3 n-3	C18:4 n-3	C20:5 n-3	C22:5 n-3	C22:6 n-3	EPA+ DHA	Total omega-3
Freshwater crawfish [97]	16	20	4		8	1	3	10	15
Scallop [97]	18	10		2	14	2	18	32	36
Common oyster [100]	36	18	3	3	11		10	21	27
Freshwater prawn [98]	19	14			16	1	7	23	24
Penaeid shrimp [50, 94]	31	34	1	1	14	1	11	25	29
Scallops [94]	21	23	4	2	16	2	21	38	46
Oysters [94]	34	32	3	7	9	1	10	19	31
Soft clams [94]	20	16	2	3	11	3	12	23	31
Surf clams [94]	29	19	1	2	11	7	8	19	30
Razor clams [94]	21	13	3	3	14	2	15	29	38
Mussels [94]	28	28	12	4	12	1	11	23	32
New Zealand Green Lipped Mussel [99]	25	21	2	3	15	1	19	34	41
Mantis shrimp edible portion [101]	26	26	2	1	13	1	16	29	32
Fleshy prawn, edible portion, [101]	28	19	1		15		15	30	31
Giant freshwater prawn edible portion [101]	29	26	1		12		5	17	18
Whiteleg shrimp edible portion [101]	34	22	2	1	12		9	21	24

In addition to the species specifically targeted for fishmeal and oil production there are other species available whose waste or by-product is converted to fishmeal and oil. These can be broken down into those currently being utilized to some extent and those with a potential for use. In some cases even though the waste is partially utilized, there is room for future growth. This can be seen in Table 6.

Crustaceans And Mollusks Fatty Acid Composition

Krill

Krill, a crustacean, is considered the last major under exploited marine species in the ocean and the largest species on earth in terms of numbers. According to the Marine Stewardship Council (MSC) certification process the biomass is estimated to be 60.3 mmt [90]. The lipid in krill is composed of both triglyceride oil and phospholipids. Depending upon how you process the krill you can obtain 3 distinct products; a whole krill oil containing both the triglyceride and phospholipid fractions, the triglyceride fraction only and the phospholipid fraction only. The phospholipid fraction can also be separated into the individual PLs. Processes currently used include solvent extraction of whole krill, drying of the krill (krill meal) followed by solvent extraction to recover both fractions separately or together, hydrolysis of the krill and wet rendering. The market is dominated by a small number of companies. Based on their patents and GRAS submissions to the US FDA the composition of these products is shown in Table 7.

Squid

Another species currently being utilized to some extent is squid. Squid is a mollusk. A small amount of squid oil is produced and offered on the omega-3 market. Squid oil is a rich source of C22:6n-3 DHA. The process used to recover the lipid is hydrolysis but extraction and rendering can also be used. Table 8 gives the fatty acid profiles of some squid extracts.

Other Crustaceans and Mollusks

Recently there have been reports that an omega-3 product is being produced from the waste of marine shrimp and there are products on the market produced from the New Zealand Green Lipped Mussel. There is no data available on the composition of the oil from the shrimp waste but Table 9 gives some indication of what the fatty acid composition would look like for other crustaceans and mollusks. It should be noted that the waste from crustaceans is approximately 60% of the total body mass.

FISHMEAL LIPID EXTRACTS

In the wet rendering process the fish are cooked and pressed to separate the liquid from the solids. The liquid fraction contains free oil, water with dissolved and suspended proteins and a middle fraction (usually an emulsion) containing phospholipids (PL), oil and water. This emulsion was always a processing problem because it interfered with the efficient separation of the oil from the aqueous phase. In fact, it was the major obstacle to recovering krill oil from the wet rendering process. The separation process therefore is designed to force the emulsion into the aqueous phase where it is then evaporated and added back to the fishmeal during the drying process.

The phospholipid content of fish flesh, from species or their by-products, used for the production of fishmeal was reported to range from 7-35% of the total lipid with an average of 17%. For whitefish species such as cod and hake, the total lipid in the flesh is very low but is composed of 80-90% phospholipid [102]. In these whitefish species most of the lipid is concentrated in the livers.

This same report indicated that for capelin, while the phospholipid content of the whole fish was 16%, it was 24% in the fishmeal produced from the capelin. Fishmeal therefore could be a rich source of marine phospholipids. A world patent application submitted in 2006 describes the process for extracting PLs from fishmeal [103]. One of the optional processes used for producing krill PLs is to first dry the krill and produce a krill meal, followed by solvent extraction. This and some of the other options have already been described [104].

SINGLE CELL OILS

Fish are unable to produce omega-3 fatty acids and therefore get them by eating organisms rich in these fatty acids, the phyto and zooplankton. Single cell oils (SCO) are the edible oils extracted from micro-organisms, which are at the bottom of the food chain. There has been interest in microbial lipids for well over 100 years, and in utilizing them and their lipids for human consumption probably since the early part of the 20th century. But it wasn't until the late 1980s when microbial oil research began to take hold with research on the production of these oils for infant formula [105]. This development paralleled developments in the production of marine oils and concentrates for the health food supplement market.

The research on SCOs dramatically increased when governments began looking for alternative sources of fuel oil. Research funds were plentiful and many start-up companies, universities and consortiums were able to access these funds to demonstrate that these SCOs could replace soy, palm and other vegetable oils that were used by the biodiesel industry. The attraction to algae was potential yield; while various crops could produce anywhere from 48 – 635 gallons of oil per acre, you could produce the equivalent of 38,000 gallons per acre with SCO production. More realistic figures put the SCO production at 4500 – 6000 gallons of oil per acre, still well above the best yielding vegetable oil source.

While the goal of producing sufficient volumes of these SCOs for fuel is still very far down the road, today, a number of organisms are used to produce SCOs and quite a few others are under investigation for the nutraceutical and animal feed markets. These materials can be the extracted lipid or the entire biomass containing the lipid. Some of these are shown in Table 10.

SEAWEEDS (MACRO ALGAE) FATTY ACID COMPOSITION

Of the total water on the earth, 97.5% is salt water and 2.5% is freshwater. However only 0.3% of the Earth's freshwater is in liquid form on the surface. Seaweeds are another potential source of lipids high in omega-3 fatty, acids among other compounds, and since the earth is covered by 75% water, there is potentially an economical reason to look at farming seaweed in the oceans instead of crops on the limited farm land. While the lipid content is low, roughly 1-2%, and seaweed can't compare to the high lipid content in microalgae, seaweed could be a potential source in the future. Today seaweeds represent about 24% of the aquaculture production and 1% of the wild capture. The raw materials are used for various food and animal feed use and for the production of carrageenan, alginate and agar [125]. Table 11 shows the composition of some red, brown and green seaweeds.

MAMMALS (SEAL)

Marine mammal oils, specifically whale and sperm whale oil, have been used over a long period of time. Once accounting for as much as 75% of the total aquatic animal oil production, today there is virtually no marine mammal oil produced. In addition to the whale oil, oil from seals, walrus, porpoise and other mammals found various uses as illuminating oils or specialty lubricants. These products are no longer used due to prohibitions on hunting these marine animals but seal hunting has remained and goes into and out of the news from time to time. In 1951 over 1 million seals were caught, but the catch dropped to a low in the late 1980 -1990 period before peaking in mid- 2000 and then dropping off again. Five countries account for most of the hunt and the harp seal is the major target. This can be seen in Table 12.

The sale of seal products has been banned in many countries who oppose any hunting of the mammals including the EU in 2009. Those who support the hunting claim that the seals are consuming too much of the available fish and thus competing with the livelihood of the fishermen and actually depleting some of the fish stocks. Canada and Norway brought a complaint before the World Trade Organization (WTO) challenging the EU ban on the sale of seal products. In June 2014 the WTO appeal board upheld the ban on the sale of seal products in the EU agreeing that the ban was "necessary_to protect public morals." The 2009 embargo applies only to commercial hunting and exempts certain indigenous groups who have traditionally hunted seals, including Canada's Inuit. In the same ruling the WTO found that the EU's application of the seal product injunction was discriminatory. It noted that "the exemption for indigenous communities did not "immediately and unconditionally" extend the same level of market access to Norway and Canada as it did to Greenland, a Danish territory whose Inuit population engages in large-scale seal hunting "closely related to those of commercial hunts." Only about 5% of both Canadian and Norwegian seal hunting is carried out by their indigenous Inuit and Sami communities, respectively [http://globalriskinsights. com/2014/ 06/08/eu-seal-case-adds-new-protectionism-to-wto/].

Table 10. Omega-3 fatty acid content of potential single cell oil sources

	% Total fatty acids										
Species	Saturates	Mono-unsaturates	C18:2 n-6	C18:3 n-3	C18:4 n-3	C20:4 n-6	C20:5 n-3	C22:5 n-6	C22:6 n-3	EPA+ DHA	Total omega-3
Nannochloropsis sp. [106]	28	31	5				35			35	35
Nannochloropsis oceanica [106]	30	29	6			3	19			19	19
Nannochloropsis oceanica [107]	37	23	10	1		4	23			23	24
Nannochloropsis. oculata [108]	36	21	10	14		5	6	1	7	13	28
Thraustochytrid sp. [109]	37	3	1				2	16	37	39	41
Schizochytrium sp. [110]	35	3			1	1	3	14	35	38	39
Schizochytrium sp. [111]	37	2					3	14	38	41	42
Schizochytrium sp. [112]	42	5					1	8	40	41	42
Schizochytrium sp. [113]	32	1	1			1	3	16	40	43	44
Schizochytrium aggregatum [108]	26	36	15	1		7	16	0	0	16	16
*Ulkenia sp.*1 [114]	39					1		11	46	46	48
Porphyridium cruentum [115]	46	4	6			22	20			20	21

	% Total fatty acids										
Species	Saturates	Mono-unsaturates	C18:2 n-6	C18:3 n-3	C18:4 n-3	C20:4 n-6	C20:5 n-3	C22:5 n-6	C22:6 n-3	EPA+ DHA	Total omega-3
Porphyridium aerugineum [115]	50	4	4			13	24			24	26
Porphyridium cruentum [117, 120]	34	3	12	1		40	7			7	8
Porphyridium cruentum [108]	36	26	1	0		17	20			20	20
Porphyridium purpureum [108]	52	9	8	9		6	7	11		7	26
Pavlova sp.[107]	23	21	2	3	6		16		11	28	33
Pavlova lutheri [108]	43	13	20	1		7	4	4	8	12	17
Pavlova lutheri [108]	37	14	9	9		5	14	6	6	20	35
Amphidinium. caterae [108]	47	10	6	3		2	15	1	17	32	37
Amphidinium sp. [100]	40	17	2	2			8		17	25	27
Chaetoceros. calcitrans [108]	42	28	5	1		1	19	5		19	24
Chlorella minutissima [108]	47	33		10		3	3	4		3	18
Chlorella minutissima [108]	20	32	6	5		6	31			31	36

Table 10. (Continued)

	% Total fatty acids										
Species	Saturates	Mono-unsaturates	C18:2 n-6	C18:3 n-3	C18:4 n-3	C20:4 n-6	C20:5 n-3	C22:5 n-6	C22:6 n-3	EPA+ DHA	Total omega-3
Chlorella minutissima [118, 119]	30	26	3		1		34			34	35
Chlorella protothecoides [116, 122]	21	65	15	1							1
Chlorella minutissima [117, 119, 121]	27	28	2			4	29			29	36
Phaeodactylum. Tricornutum [108]	21	44	4	1		3	21	6	1	22	28
Phaeodactylum tricornutum [107, 119]	28	29	2		3	2	28	1	4	32	35
Rhodomonas baltica [107]	17	4	12	12	5		4	2		4	22
Isochrysis galbana [100, 117]	28	14	2		11		25		11	36	47
Isochrysis galbana [108]	38	22	4	13		1	17	1	4	20	34
Isochrysis galbana [107]	20	16	7	4	13		1	1	16	17	33
Yarrowia lipolytica [123]	6	7	19	4	2		36			36	43
Thraustochytrium aureum [100]	11	16	2	2		3			52	52	54
Skeletonema costanum [100]	27	13	1		6		41		7	48	54
Parietochloris incisa [118]	13	18	17	2		43	1			1	3

	% Total fatty acids										
Species	Saturates	Mono-unsaturates	C18:2 n-6	C18:3 n-3	C18:4 n-3	C20:4 n-6	C20:5 n-3	C22:5 n-6	C22:6 n-3	EPA+ DHA	Total omega-3
Desmarestia acculeata [118]	16	9	6	2	16	19	19			19	56
Chrysophyta salina [108]	37	27	20	3		4	8	1		8	12
Crypthecodinium cohinii [108]	34	40	2	1		1		2	20	20	23
Crypthecodinium cohnii [113] ok	38	17	1						42	42	42
Cryptomonas sp. [108]	45	21	1	2		3	17	1	10	27	29
Monodus subterraneus [108]	20	28	2			14	34	1		34	36
Mortierella alpina [81]	31	10	14			35					1
Mortierella elongata [117]	9	18	12			16	15			15	15
Mortierella alpina [124]	32	7	9			44					1
Prorocentrum minimum [108]	57	6	6	11		3	9	3	6	15	28
Thalassiosira. pseudonana [108, 120]	40	24	3	1		9	11	7	7	17	25
Thrautocytrium aureum [108]	16	22	11	15		12	5	4	16	21	40

Table 11. Fatty acid content of some red, brown and green algae [126]

Species	Saturates	Mono-unsaturates	C16:4 n-3	C18:2 n-6	C18:3 n-3	C18:4 n-3	C20:4 n-6	C20:5 n-3	Total omega-3
	% of Total fatty acids								
RED ALGAE									
Porphyra yezoensis	27	11		2		1	2	53	54
Odonthalia dentata	30	5		2	3	3	9	43	51
Laurencia obtuse	20	5	2	2	2	2	5	48	56
Ceramium rubrum	26	11		3	3	4	8	26	36
Batrachospermum moniliforme	26	14		2	1	1	9	42	44
BROWN ALGAE									
Laminaria saccharin	14	8		4	10	20	9	28	62
Alaria esculenta	15	7		4	11	28	12	18	57
Fucus spiralis	29	19		7	7	7	14	7	40
Pelvetia canaliculata	17	30		10	3	1	14	5	9
Chondrus crispus	20	11	3	4	6	6	13	26	45
Scytosiphon lomentaria	20	11		7	8	19	8	23	50
Fucus vesiculosus	27	24		10	8	7	15	14	29
GREEN ALGAE									
Cladophora rupestris	21	9	15		2	3	3	6	26
Ulva lactuca	18	9	17		17	24	1	2	60
Enteromorpha intestinalis	13	9	16	6	21	17	1	2	56
Enteromorpha compressa	28	15	7	12	14	6	2	2	29

Table 12. Species of seal hunted for various products including seal oil

	Country and %	10 Year Average Landings, numbers
Harp seal, 68% of the hunt	Canada 65%, Greenland 27%, Norway %, Russian Federation 3%	281,534
Ringed seal, 18% of the hunt	Greenland 95%, Russian Federation 5%	74,280
So. African Fur Seal, 12% of the hunt	Namibia 100%	49,400
Northern Fur Seal, 0.6% of the hunt	Russian Federation, 100%	2,281
Hooded Fur Seal, 0.8% of the hunt	Greenland 100%	3,476
Others, 1% of the hunt	Other countries	4,083
Totals		415,054

Seal oil has been promoted as a rich source of omega-3 fatty acids and seal oil capsules are sold in the countries where this is permitted.

Table 13 compares the fatty acid composition of seal oil or the blubber from some of the seals that are hunted.

Genetically Modified Plant Oils

With the growth of the omega-3 market over the past 30+ years it was no surprise to see the non-fish oil groups join the research. For a very long time fish oil was considered the least expensive oil on the commodity market because of the polyunsaturated fatty acids (PUFA). The oil was not suitable for the edible market (primarily margarines, shortening and other baking fats) because the PUFA tended to oxidize and cause rancid and or fishy flavors in foods to which they were added. It was therefore necessary to partially hydrogenate the marine oils to reduce or eliminate these PUFA. The PUFA, of course, were primarily the long chain omega-3 fatty acids. Vegetable oils also have omega-3s but they were the shorter chain length fatty acids but even they caused rancid flavors in foods. Generally, everyone was pursuing ways to remove or reduce these omega-3 fatty acids in their oils.

The hydrogenation process was very effective in eliminating the problem fatty acids but in the process *trans* fatty acids were formed. Eventually it was determined that these *trans* fatty acids were not healthy when consumed and legislation in various countries including the USA has now banned or is in the process of banning them. This has effectively reduced the hydrogenation market quite substantially and caused the shift in the marine oil market towards aquaculture where the omega-3 fatty acids are essential.

Table 13. Omega-3 fatty acid content of the lipid from several species of seal

	% Total fatty acids									
Species	Satu-rates	Mono-unsaturates	C18:2 n-6	C18:3 n-3	C18:4 n-3	C20:4 n-6	C20:5 n-3	C22:5 n-6	C22:6 n-3	EPA+ DHA	Total omega-3
Seal oil, nei [127]	14	49	2	1		1	8	4	9	17	24
Hooded seal (female) blubber [128]	12	73	3				3		3	6	7
Leopard seal blubber [128]	15	62	2	1	2		5	3	8	13	19
Crab eater seal blubber [128]	17	54	3	1	2		6	4	13	19	26
Harbor seal blubber [128]	11	69	1		1		6	4	8	13	19
Alaska fur seal blubber [128]	20	35	9				5		3	9	9
So. American fur seal [128]	30	63									6
Seal oil nei [129]	13	48	1	1			7	3	7	14	21
Seal oil nei [130]	15	62	2		1		6	4	7	13	19
Seal Oil nei [131]	13	48	2	1	4		7	4	11	18	26
Harbor seal(male) blubber [132]	11	59	1		1	1	7	8	13	19	28
Harbor seal (female) blubber [132]	13	47	1		1	1	11	8	17	27	36
Ribbon seal (male) blubber [132]	10	52	1		1	1	8	8	17	26	35
Ribbon seal (female) blubbe r [132]	14	51	1	1	1	1	8	7	15	23	32
Ringed seal (male) blubber [132]	10	43	1	1	1		12	12	18	30	44
Ringed seal (female) blubber [132]	7	41	1		1		11	15	26	37	53
Bearded seal (male) blubber [132]	14	40	1		1	1	14	10	12	26	38
Bearded seal (female) blubber [132]	17	50	1		1	1	9	5	13	23	30

Table 14. The fatty acid composition of some transgenic plants

	% Total fatty acids									
	Saturates	Monounsaturates	C18:2 n-6	C18:3 n-3	C18:3 n-6	C18:4 n-3	C20:4 n-6	C20:5 n-3	C22:5 n-3	C22:6 n-3
High SDA soybean oil [134]	17	15	21	10	7	23				
Arabidopsis thaliana [135]	13	35	26	13		1	1	2		
Brassica juncea [136]	8	20	15	4	28	3	8	4		
Arabidopsis thaliana [137]	11	34	18	11	11	3	3	3		
Camelina satvia [142]	13	20	8	29		9		3	1	12
Camelina satvia [142]	13	9	10	3	1	9		3	1	12
Arabidopsis sp. [143]	18	15	4	30		6		2	2	15
Camelina satvia EPA line[144] [1]	15	9	18	13	2	1	2	23	1	
Camelina satvia DHA line[144] [1]	15	13	19	12	4	3	2	11	2	6

[1] Total lipid.

As the omega-3 market for human food consumption began to grow quite rapidly, it fostered research to find ways to genetically modify the plant biochemistry so that it could effectively produce these marine fatty acids within the oilseeds. Projections for continued growth in the omega-3 and aquaculture markets are causing concerns about insufficient supplies of suitable marine oils and what better way to get around this problem than to be able to plant more and more acres of genetically modified (GM) plants with the long chain PUFA found in fish. The production of very long chain PUFA in land plants has been a long-standing goal of bioengineers around the world. The first demonstrations of LC-PUFA production were published in 2004 and showed EPA and ARA production in leaf and seed [133]. One of the first successes was the Monsanto high Stearadonic acid (SDA) soybean oil which received Generally Recognized as Safe (GRAS) status by the US Food and Drug Administration (USFDA) in 2009 [134]. Since then, global research at various institutions has achieved the modification of various oilseeds so that they produce either EPA or DHA. The first demonstrations of DHA production in seed were published soon after. Subsequent work resulted in increasing levels of production, particularly for EPA. The first report of production of fish oil-like levels of DHA in seed was published in 2012. Progress has been extensively reviewed in recent years [135-141].

Just 3 years ago, it was suggested that actual commercial production of transgenic plants containing levels of EPA and DHA similar to fish oil was at least 10 years down the road. In 2014 the UK government gave their approval for commercial test plots to grow transgenic *camelina* with relatively high levels of EPA and DHA [145]. Harvesting of the seeds from these test plots is expected in august 2014.

Some of these transgenic lines can be seen in Table 14.

Conclusion

In 1996 a conference was held in Cape Town South Africa. One of the sessions covered the major issue for the marine oil industry at the time. If *trans* fatty acids are banned, what are we going to do with 1 million tons of fish oil since the market was primarily for hydrogenation and *trans* fatty acids are produced during the hydrogenation process? In 2012 another conference was held in Boston, Massachusetts USA. One of the themes of that conference was where are we going to get sufficient marine oils to supply the growing omega 3 food and health food supplement market? In 2012 very little oil was going into the hydrogenation market with most being used in the aquaculture industry.

It's quite apparent from various reports and studies that the demand for fish and fish products is approaching the limits of supply from the oceans. Various reports indicate that to cover this shortfall the supply of fish must come from the aquaculture segment of the industry. However there is a problem; some of the major aquaculture species require marine proteins and lipids to supply the essential nutrients in their feeds and these are currently supplied by wild caught fish. As demand exceeds supply, prices increase and this has offered incentives to find new raw material sources. Global research is attempting to substitute various animal, plant and insect proteins and oils for the marine proteins and oils. I prefer the word extend rather than substitute since we will always have marine proteins and oils available. Research is also evaluating micro and macro algae products as well as transgenic plant materials for both the oils, proteins and combined in the whole biomass. One of the major issues relates to diluting out the omega-3 in the marine lipids and replacing them with omega-6 from non-marine sources. This could neutralize the omega-3 benefits of eating fish.

The imbalance in supply and demand has also produced opportunities to recover valuable lipids and proteins from the waste or by-products of edible fish processing. In the past, these by-products were mostly discarded in landfills or disposed of at sea before the fishing vessel returned to port. Pollock oil, for example was recovered on board processing vessels but then burned as fuel. Today it is beginning to appear in omega-3 health food supplements. We must remember that edible fish generate on average about 50% waste when the fish are processed, shrimp can generate as much as 60-65% waste.

As these products enter the marine oil market, data on the actual fatty acid composition of the oil becomes very important. Generally, researchers are simply doing a Bligh and Dyer total lipid extract and then analyzing the fatty acid composition of the extracted total lipid. Unfortunately this type of extract doesn't really express the fatty acid profile of an oil that could be produced because some of the lipid would go with the protein fraction via the aqueous phase of the process. Krill processing is the exception since the lipid is generally solvent extracted from the dried biomass and thus you get the phospholipid fraction dissolved in the neutral lipids. It has been suggested that researchers begin to evaluate the oil produced by simply steam cooking the fish or waste and squeezing out the oil. This can be done in a "boil in the bag" type system. Obviously it is not as convenient as the B&D method but the data would go a long way in generating interest from the health food supplement industry and perhaps open up new markets for fishery by-products. Some of this is already being done with shrimp, squid and aquaculture by-products.

The production of microalgae rich in omega-3 marine lipids continues to grow for both the animal feed and human health food market. In some cases, companies are simply producing the biomass and then drying it into an oily cake. This is then being fed to fish, pets and laying hens for omega-3 eggs. The drying method eliminates the issue of recovering the oil fraction and takes advantage of both the protein and lipid fractions in one product. However, if the oil content of the biomass is very high there is a possibility of spontaneous combustion and or oxidation of the lipids if the biomass is not stabilized with antioxidants.

Microalgae production is growing. It is still very expensive compared to fish proteins and oils but as the price of the fish proteins and oils increases and the price of the microalgae decreases, it will become more attractive especially in specialty markets.

Not too long ago transgenic plants, seemed to be about 10 years down the road before reaching commercial viability. Today, there is a commercial sized test plot of transgenic *camelina satvia* being grown in the UK. The seeds were planted in May 2014 and the crop will be harvested in August 2014. Table 14 shows several transgenic lines for *camelina satvia,* with EPA and DHA. However it is not clear at this time what the harvested seeds will contain. Initially the protein and oil will be targeted for the aquaculture market but eventually they could go into the food and food supplement market if the market can reconcile the GMO issues. Work in this area continues and the results will be quite interesting in the next few years.

Looking forward, we will see more and more of the "industrial fish" being used for human consumption and more and more of the by-products recovered for use in the production of marine proteins and oils. Today, about 25-35% of the raw materials used for the production of marine proteins and oils comes from by-products. When you consider that the targeted fishmeal and oil species only represent about 15-20% of the total fish landings, it opens up a potentially large raw material supply pool of by-product that could come from the waste. And since the same issues relate to the aquaculture segment of the market, the potential for additional raw materials from that growing segment is large. It doesn't require large fishmeal plants to recover oil from these by-products. Small scale hydrolysis (silage) plants located adjacent to salmon farming operations and wild salmon processing plants are producing suitable omega-3 oils for the health food supplement market today.

Krill is considered a major unexploited biomass that is not being fished anywhere near the sustainability limits. However krill is also the food for whales, penguins, seabirds and fish. Taking food away from baby penguins, whales or seabirds is an emotional issue and even approaching the sustainable limits for this species will generate a firestorm from environmental groups. Krill oil is popular in the health food supplement market, is relatively expensive and while the market will continue to grow it will remain a specialty high value product.

REFERENCES

[1] FAO. FishStat J Release: 2.0.0 a tool for fishery statistics analysis, at http://www.fao.org/fishery/statistics/software/fishstatj/cn (2014).

[2] Anonymous. *Global Aquaculture Advocate* 16, 16 (2013).

[3] J. Shepherd, *World Agriculture* 3, 11 (2012).

[4] Anonymous, Book of Tobit Chapter 6. *The Bible, at* http://www.catholic.org/bible/book.php?id=17&bible_chapter=6 (2014).

[5] Robert I. Curtis, *The Classical Journal*, 78, 232 at http://ancienthistory.about.com/od/romanfood/g/garum.htm (1983).

[6] Ilona Gerbakher, *Agathai Quarterly Journal* 2, 5 at http://www.mortarboardatucla.org/uploads/4/7/8/9/4789362/issue_201.pdf (2011).

[7] K. J. Whittle. Marine Organisms as Food, Forage, Industrial, and Medical Products, in Ed. Patrick Safran. *Fisheries and Aquaculture* VOL. I, pp 144-177, in *Encyclopedia of Life Support Systems (EOLSS)*, Developed under the Auspices of the UNESCO, Eolss Publishers, UK, [http://www.eolss.net] (2009).

[8] Charles H. Stevenson, *US Fish Commission Report from 1902* pages 177-279. Washington Government Printing Office at https://archive.org/stream/aquaticproductsi00stev#page/n1/mode/2up (1903).

[9] FAO, *FAO Fisheries Technical Paper 142 Rev 1*, Food and Agriculture Organization of the United Nations, Rome 63 pages (1986).

[10] D. L. Alverson , M. K. Freeberg, S. A. Murawski and J. G. Pope, *FAO Fisheries Technical Paper No 339* Food and Agriculture Organization of the United Nations , Rome (1996).

[11] Kieran Kelleher, 2005, *FAO Fisheries Technical Paper 470*. Food and Agriculture Organization of the United Nations, Rome 154 pages (2005).

[12] Achim Steiner, UNEP talk at Save Food Congress, Dusseldorf Germany at http://www.unep.org/NewsCentre/default.aspx?ArticleID= 10858 &DocumentID=2790 , May 7, 2014

[13] Anthony P. Bimbo, Processing of marine oils, in Ed Breivik, Harald *Long-chain omega-3 specialty oils.* Bridgewater, Oily Press pages 77–109, (2007).

[14] Hordur Kristinsson, Value Added Utilization of Seafood Processing By-Products. Paper presented at the 2010 Atlantic Fisheries Technology Conference, St. Johns Newfoundland, (2010).

[15] Anthony P. Bimbo, Rendering. In Ed. Fereidoon Shahidi. *Bailey's Industrial Oil & Fat Products 6th edition Vol 6* pp.57-102, John Wiley & Sons, Hoboken NJ USA, (2005).

[16] Malcolm Windsor, *Torry Advisory Note No. 39*, Torry Research Station, Aberdeen, Scotland, UK , (1969).

[17] John Spinelli, , Virginia F. Stout and William B. Nilsson. United States Patent 4,692,280, September 8, 1987.

[18] Virginia Stout and John Spinelli. United States Patent 4,675,132, June 23, 1987.

[19] Hordur G. Kristinsson, and Demir Necla, Functional Fish Protein Ingredients from Fish Species of Warm, and Temperate Waters: Comparison of Acid-and Alkali Aided Processing vs. Conventional Surimi Processing, in Ed. Peter J. Bechtel *Advances in Seafood Byproducts 2002 Conference Proceedings*, Alaska Sea Grant College Program, University of Alaska Fairbanks), (2003).

[20] Hultin, Herbert O., Stephen D. Kelleher,Yuming Feng, Mark P. Richards, Hordur Kristinsson, Ingrid Vndeland, Giiteborg, and Shuming Ke, *United States Patent,* 7,556,835, July 7, 2009.

[21] The Sustainable Fisheries Partnership 2014. *Small Pelagics: SFP Fisheries Sustainability Overview 2014* at http://cmsdevelopment.sustainablefish.org.s3.amazonaws.com/2014/06/17/Small_Pelagics_Sector_Report_2014_-_FINAL-396e5e21.pdf (2014).

[22] FAO, *The state of world fisheries and agriculture; opportunities and challenges*, Food and Agriculture Organization of the United Nations Rome 244 pages, (2014).

[23] CCAMLR, *CCAMLR Statistical Bulletin, Vol. 26 (1970-2013),* at https://www.ccamlr.org/en/document/data/ccamlr-statistical-bulletin-vol-26, (2014).

[24] Oil World. *Global analysis of all major oilseeds, oils and oilmeals supply, demand and price outlook*, Ed. Thomas Mielke, ISTAMielke GmbH, Hamburg, (2014).

[25] Anthony P. Bimbo, Processing of marine oils, in Ed. Harald Breivik, *Long-chain omega-3 specialty oils.* Bridgewater, Oily Press pages 77 - 109. (2007).

[26] IFFO AnnualYearbook of Data at http://www.iffo.net/iffoupdate (2013).

[27] GOED, Global supply and demand trends in omega-3 fish oils , presentation at the IFFO Market Forum April 17, Miami Florida, at http://portal.sliderocket.com/GOEDomega3/IFFO-Miami-Meeting-2012 (2012).

[28] GOED, Global supply and demand trends in omega3 fish oils' presentation at the IFFO Market Forum April 17 London, UK at http://www.iffo.net/members-area/2014-london-workshop-session and market-forum-iii (2014).

[29] E. G. Bligh and W. J. Dyer, *Can. J. Biochem. Physiol.,* 37, 20 (1959).

[30] Anthony P. Bimbo, *Inform* 9, 473 (1998).

[31] R. G. Ackman, Fish oils, in Ed. Fereidoon Shahidi, *Bailey's Industrial Oil and Fat Products, Sixth Edition.* Hoboken, Wiley - Interscience pages 279 – 317 (2005).

[32] Angélica Ganga, Susana Nieto, Julio Sanhuez, Claudio Romo, Hernán Speisky and Alfonso Valenzuela, *JAOCS* 75, 733 (1998).

[33] O. Cornejo, personal communication (2012).

[34] Kajal Chakraborty, P. Vijayagopal, Rekha D. Chakraborty and K.K Vijayan, *Food Chem.* 120, 433 (2010).

[35] Chitra R.S Som , *Bioactivity Profile of Polyunsaturated Fatty acid extracts from Sardinella longiceps and Sardinella fimbriata -A Comparative Study.* Ph. D. Cochin University Of Science And Technology (2010).

[36] D. W. Liyanage, D. R. C Wijesundera and T. W. Wikramanayake, *Ceylon J. Med. Sci.,* 32, 23 (1989).

[37] A. Khoddami, A. A. Ariffin, J. Bakar, S. Ravichandran and H.M. Ghazali, *World Applied Sci. J.* 7,127 (2009).

[38] Y. Ando, K. Nishimura, N. Aoyanagi and T. Takagi, *JAOCS* 69, 417 (1992).

[39] Kenji Hayashi, Hideki Kishimura, *Bulletin of the faculty of fisheries Hokkaido University*, 44, 24-31, (1993), at http://eprints2008.lib.hokudai.ac.jp/dspace/bitstream/2115/24106/1/44(1)_P24-31.pdf (1993).

[40] Toru Takagi, personal communication, (1993).

[41] M. B. Hale, *Marine Fisheries Review* 46, 19 (1984).
[42] A. Bimbo, *JAOCS* 66,1717 (1989).
[43] A. Bimbo, personal data (2011).
[44] Charmian J. O'Connor , Sagar, R Katvi and Qiong Chen, A survey of omega-3 fatty acids in common New Zealand seafood, in Ed. Charmian J O'Connor and Lawrence Eyres. *Handbook of Australasian edible oils,* Auckland , Oils and Fats Specialist Group of NZIC 297 pages (2007).
[45] P. D. Nichols, Fish oil sources in Ed. Harald Breivik *Long Chain Omega-3 Specialty Oils*. Bridgewater, The Oily Press, pages 23-42 (2007).
[46] S. Sigurgisladottir and H. Palmadottir, *JAOCS*, 70, 1081 (1993).
[47] P.G. Dunne, D. Cronin, A. Martine, H. Brennan and T.R. Gormley, *J. Fisheries Sciences* 4, 269 (2010).
[48] P. Vlieg and D.R. Body, *New Zealand J. Marine Freshwater Res.* 22, 151 (1988).
[49] Jakobsen , Jan Vidar Fish trial with crude and carbon filtered fish oils from Denmark and Iceland. Nor Aqua Innovation AS Research Report 2001-2, 12 pages, at http://www.iffo.net/downloads/Research%20 reports/IFOMA%201978-2001/2001/Fish%20trials%20with%20crude%20and%20carbon%20filtered%20fish%20oils%202001-2.pdf (2001).
[50] S.J. Iverson, K.J. Frost and S.L. C. Lang, *Mar. Ecol. Prog. Ser.* 241, 161 (2002).
[51] Sevim Kose, personal communication (2011).
[52] B. Tufan, S. Koral and S. Kose, *Internat. J. Food Sci. Technol.* 46, 800 (2011).
[53] A. Oksuz and A. Ozyılmaz, *Turkish J. Fish. Aq. Sci.* 10, 381 (2010).
[54] G. Ustiin, A. Akova and L. Dandik, *JAOCS*, 73, 389 (1996).
[55] J. V. Visentainer , M. D'Addio Noffs, P. de Oliveira Carvalho, V.V. de Almeida , C. C. de Oliveira, N.E. de Souzao, *JAOCS* 84, 543 (2007).
[56] N. Marisa and C. Litz, *Ecology of the Northern Subpopulation of Northern Anchovy (Engraulis mordax) in the California Current Large Marine Ecosystem* M Sc. Oregon State University, (2008).
[57] M. D. Huynh, D.D. Kitts, C. Hu and A.W. Trites, *Comparative Biochem. Physiol.* 146, 504 (2007).
[58] http://slism.com/calorie/110008/ Atlantic Horse Mackerel Calories and Quick Look At Nutrition Facts (2014).
[59] http://slism.com/calorie/110003 Japanese Horse Mackerel Calories and Quick Look At Nutrition Facts (2014).

[60] K. Nisa and K. Asadullah, *Iranian J. Fish. Sci.* 10, 67 (2011).
[61] K. Osako, H. Saito, M.A. Hossain, K. Kuwahara and A. Okamoto, *Lipids*, 41, 713 (2006).
[62] Zied Khiari , *Functional and bioactive components from mackerel (Scomber scombrus) and blue whiting (Micromesistius poutassou) processing waste* Ph. D. Dublin Institute of Technology (2010).
[63] M.B. Hale and T. Brown, *Marine Fish. Rev.* 45, 4 (1983).
[64] D. Fernandez-Jover, J.A. Lopez Jimenez, P. Sanchez-Jerez, J. Bayle-Sempere, F. Gimenez-Casalduero, F.J. Martinez Lopez and T. Dempster, *Mar. Environ. Res.* 63, 1 (2007).
[65] M. Stancheva, B. Galunska, A.D Dobreva and A. Merdzhanova, *Grasas y Aceites*, 63, 152 (2012).
[66] L.T.C. Huang, P. Bulbul, C. Wen, R.H. Glew and F.A. Ayaz, *J. Food Sci.* 77, 512 (2012).
[67] J.L. Guil-Guerrero and E.H. Belarbi, *JAOCS*, 78, 477 (2001).
[68] W. Kolanowski, *Internat. J. Food Properties*, 13, 498 (2010).
[69] Sandro Lane, personal communication (2012).
[70] Alexandra C.M Oliveira, Trina J. Lapis, Tobias Popp, Brian Himelbloom and Scott Smiley, The Chemical Composition and oxidative stability of Alaska commercial salmon oils. in Ed. Peter J Bechtel and Scott Smiley, *A Sustainable Future: Fish Processing Byproducts.* Fairbanks, Alaska Sea Grant College Program, Univ of Alaska pages 241-257 (2010).
[71] T. van Vliet and M.B. Katan, *Am. J. Clin. Nutr.* 51, 1 (1990).
[72] Siri Tømmerås, *Fat, fatty acids and fat soluble nutrients in fillet of farmed and wild Atlantic salmon (Salmo salar L.),* MSc University of Tromso UIT at http://munin.uit.no/bitstream/handle/10037/3475/thesis.pdf?sequence=2 (2011).
[73] J. Cowger, personal communication (2009).
[74] A.C.M Oliveira, *Purification of pollock oil using short path distillation.* Pollock conservation cooperative research center final report, http://www.sfos.uaf.edu/pcc/projects/08/oliveira/Purification_of_pollock_oil_FINAL_report_Oliveira_2010.pdf (2010).
[75] P. D. Nichols , P. Virtue, B. D. Mooney, N. G. Elliott, and G. K. Yearsley, *Seafood the good food: the oil content and composition of Australian commercial fishes, shellfishes and crustaceans*, Fisheries Research and Development Corporation Report, 200 pages (1998).
[76] S. Soltan and R.A. Gibson, *Asia Pac. J. Clin. Nutr.* 17, 385 (2008).
[77] E. Méndez, *JAOCS*, 74, 1173 (1997).

[78] Puleva Biotech, GRAS notification- Eupoly-EPA and Eupoly-DHA derived from fish oils. GRN 00193 at http://www.accessdata.fda.gov/scripts/fcn/gras_notices/grn000193.pdf (2006).

[79] A. Khoddami, A.A. Ariffin, J. Bakar and H.M. Ghazali, *African J. Biotechnol.* 11, 1683 (2012).

[80] Clover Corporation Ltd., GRAS notification- Hi DHA tuna oil GRN 0097, at http://www.accessdata.fda.gov/scripts/fcn/gras_notices/203487a.pdf (2001).

[81] Ross Laboratories Div.,Abbott Laboratories GRAS notification- GRAS determination for docosahexaenoic acid rich oil derived from tuna and arachidonic acid rich oil derived from *mortierella alpina,* GRN 0094 at http://www.accessdata.fda.gov/scripts/fcn/gras_notices/grn000094A.pdf (2001).

[82] P. D. Nichols, "Fish oil sources" in Ed. H. Breivik, *Long Chain Omega-3 Specialty Oils*. Bridgewater, The Oily Press, pages 23-42 (2007).

[83] Pesquera Pacific Star, personal communication (2005).

[84] B.T. Ho and D.R. Paul, *Internat. Food Res. J.* 16, 501 (2009).

[85] M. Pauga, *The effects of consuming farmed salmon compared to salmon oil capsules on long chain omega 3 fatty acids and selenium status in humans.* MSc thesis Massey University, New Zealand (2009).

[86] N. Shirai, "Fish Sources of Various Lipids Including n-3 Polyunsaturated Fatty Acids and their dietary effects", in Ed. E.M. Hernandez and M. Hosokawa, *Omega-3 Oils Applications in Functional Foods*. Urbana AOCS Press, pages 61-71 (2011).

[87] J.A. Nettleton, Fatty acids in cultivated and wild fish. In IIFET (International Institute of Fisheries Economics & Trade), *Microbehavior and macroresults: proceedings of the tenth biennial conference of the International Institute of Fisheries Economics and Trade presentations*, Corvallis, OR 10-14 July 2000, at http://oregonstate.edu/dept/iifet/2000/papers/nettleton2 (2000).

[88] Anthony Bimbo, personal information, (1994).

[89] A.M. Abouel-Yazeed, *J. Arabian Aquacult. Soc.* 8, 283 (2013).

[90] Marine Stewardship Council (MSC), Aker Biomarine Antarctic Krill MSC Status at http://www.msc.org/track-a-fishery/fisheries-in-the-program/certified/southern-ocean/aker-biomarine-antarctic-krill (2010).

[91] Aker Biomarine Antarctic AS GRAS notification- high phospholipid krill oil GRN000371 at http://www.accessdata.fda.gov/scripts/fcn/gras_notices/GRN000371.pdf (2010).

[92] Neptune Technologies & Bioresources GRAS notification - high phospholipid krill oil GRN 000242 at http://www.accessdata.fda.gov/scripts/fcn/gras_notices/grn000242.pdf (2008).
[93] D. Sclabos Katevas, T. Guerra, R. Raul, C. Lay, M. Mario, *United States Patent Application* 201110224450 Al, September 15, (2011).
[94] J.D. Joseph, "Distribution and composition of lipids in marine invertebrates" in Ed. R.G. Ackman, *Marine Biogenic Lipids, Fats and OilsVolume II* e CRC Press Inc Boca Raton. Pages 49-143 (1989).
[95] P. Adlercreutz and A.M. Lyberg, *International Patent Application* WO 2008/133573 Al. November 6 (2008).
[96] R. Chedoloh, T.T Karrila and P. Pakdeechanuan, *Internat. Food Res. J.* 18, 783 (2011).
[97] V. Öhrvik, A. von Malmborg, I. Mattisson, S. Wretling and C. Åstrand. Fish, shellfish and fish products- analysis of LivsmedelsVerket National Food Agency nutrients Rapport 1 – 2012 Appendix III, Sweden 47 pages (2012).
[98] A. Hanan, T. El-Din, M.M. Habashy and H.M. Sultan, *World J. Zoology* 4, 205 (2009).
[99] K. Murphy, J. Neil, J. Mann, and A.J. Sinclair, *Asia Pacific J Clin. Nutr.* 12, 50 (2003).
[100] F. Shahidi, "Marine oils from seafood waste" in Ed. F. Shahidi, *Maximizing the value of marine by-products*, CRC Press Boca Raton, pages 258-278 (2007).
[101] G. Li, A.J. Sinclair and J.D. Li, *J. Agric. Food Chem.* 59, 1871 (2011).
[102] J. Opstvedt, *IFOMA Technical Bulletin No. 22*. International Fishmeal and Fish Oil Organization, London UK, at http://www.iffo.net/animal-feeding (1985).
[103] M. Schneider and E. Lovaas, WO 2006/106325 Al, October 12 (2006).
[104] A.P. Bimbo, "Processing of marine oils" in Ed. Harald Breivik, *Long-chain omega-3 specialty oils.* Bridgewater, Oily Press pages 77–109 (2007).
[105] C. Ratledge, "Single Cell Oils for the 21st Century" in Ed. Z. Cohen and C. Ratledge. *Single Cell Oils* pages 1-20, AOCS Press Champaign (2005).
[106] J.H. Bae and S.B. Hur, *Fish Aquat. Sci.* 14, 323 (2011).
[107] V. Patil, T. Kallqvist, E. Olsen, G. Vogt and H.R. Gislerød, *Aquacult. Int.* 15, 1 (2007).
[108] R. Vazhappilly and F.A Chen, *JAOCS* 75, 393 (1998).

[109] M.R. Miller, P.D. Nichols and C.G. Carter, *Nutrition Res. Rev.* 21, 85 (2008).
[110] Martek, GRAS notification-DHA algal oil derived from Schizochytrium sp. GRN 00137, at http://www.accessdata.fda.gov/scripts/ fcn/gras_notices/706545A.PDF (2003).
[111] S.D. Doughman, S. Krupanidhi and C.B. Sanjeevi, *Current Diabetes Rev.* 3, 198 (2007).
[112] Ocean Nutrition Canada DHA rich algal oil from *Schizochytrium sp.* ONC T18, A submission to the UK Food Standards Agency requesting consideration of substantial equivalence to DHA-rich algal oil from *Schizochytrium sp.* authorized in accordance with Regulation (EC) No. 258/97 Submitted 10th October 2011, at http://www.food.gov.uk/ multimedia/pdfs/dharich (2011).
[113] A.S. Ryan, M.A. Keske, J.P. Hoffman and E.B. Nelson, *American J. Therapeutics* 16, 183 (2009).
[114] Lonza GRAS notification - Ulkenia DHA oil derived from ulkenia sp. GRN 000319 at http://www.accessdata.fda.gov/scripts/fcn/gras_notices/GRN000319.pdf (2010).
[115] G.L. K1yacbko-Gurvlch, J. Doucha, J. Kopezkil, I. E Ryabykh and V.E Semeneoko, *Russian J. Plant Physiol.* 41, 281 (1994).
[116] Z. Cohen and I. Khozin-Goldberg, "Searching for PUFA-Rich Microalgae" in Ed. Z. Cohen and C. Ratledge. *Single Cell Oils* pages 53-72 AOCS Press Champaign (2005).
[117] C. Ratledge and S. Hopkins, "Lipids from microbial sources" in Ed. F.D. Gunstone. *Modifying lipids for use in food* pp 80–113 Woodhead Publishing Limited Cambridge (2006).
[118] A. Seto, H.L Wang and C.W. Hesseltine, *JAOCS* 61, 892 (1984).
[119] N. Sultana and M.A. Hossain, *Indian J. Fish.* 36, 307 (1989).
[120] C. Bigogno, I. Khozin-Goldberg, S. Boussiba, A. Vonshaka, Z. Cohen, *Phytochem.* 60, 497 (2002).
[121] Q. Hu, M. Sommerfeld, E. Jarvis, M. Ghirardi, M. Posewitz, M. Seibert and A.L. Darzins, *The Plant J.* 54, 621 (2008).
[122] Solazyme, GRAS Application 384 Algalin Oil at http://www.fda.gov/ ucm/groups/fdagov-public/@fdagov-foods-gen/documents/document/ucm265962.pdf (2011).
[123] DuPont, GRAS notice- EPA rich triglyceride oil GRN 0355. at http://www.accessdata.fda.gov/scripts/fcn/gras_notices/GRN000355.pdf (2010).

[124] EFSA. Scientific Opinion of the Panel on Dietetic Products Nutrition and Allergies on a request from the European Commission on the safety of `fungal oil from *Mortierella alpina*`. *The EFSA Journal* 770, 1 (2008).

[125] FAO, *FAO Fisheries Technical Paper 441*. Food and Agriculture Organization of the UN, Rome 105 pages (2003).

[126] M. Kayama, S. Araki and S. Sato, "Lipids of Marine Plants" in Ed. R.G. Ackman, *Marine Biogenic Lipids, Fats and OilsVolume II*. CRC Press Inc Boca Raton. Pages 3-48 (1989).

[127] T.M. Madland, T. Björkkjær, L.A. Brunborg, L. Fröyland, A. Berstad and J.G. Brun, *J. Rheumatol.* 33, 307 (2006).

[128] R.G. Ackman and F. Lamothe, "Marine Mammals" in Ed. R.G. Ackman, *Marine Biogenic Lipids, Fats and OilsVolume II*. CRC Press Inc Boca Raton. Pages 179-381 (1989).

[129] T. Bjørkkjær, L.A. Brunborg, G. Arslan, R.A. Lind, J.G. Brun, M. Valen, B. Klementsen, A. Berstad and L. Frøyland, *Scand. J. Gastroenterol.* 11, 1088 (2004).

[130] M. Schreiner, H.W. Hulan, E. Razzazi-Fazeli, J. Bohm and C. Iben, *Poultry Sci.* 83, 462 (2004).

[131] J. Brox , K. Olaussen, B. Osterud, E.O. Elvevoll, E. Bjornstad, T. Brenn, G. Brattebo and H. Iversen, *Lipids* 36, 7 (2001).

[132] F. Shahidi and Y. Zhong, "Marine Mammal Oils" in Ed. F. Shahidi, *Bailey Industrial Oil and Fat Products 6th Edition* Hoboken, Wiley - Interscience pages 259 – 278 (2005).

[133] M. Venegas-Calerón, O. Sayanova, J.A. Napier, *Progress Lipid Res.* 49, 108 (2010).

[134] Monsanto, GRAS notice- stearidonic (SDA) omega-3 soybean oil GRN 00283 at http://www.accessdata.fda.gov/scripts/fcn/gras_notices/grn000283.pdf (2009).

[135] S.S. Robert, S.P. Singh, X.R. Zhou, J.R. Petrie, S.I. Blackburn, *Functional Plant Biol.* 32, 473 (2005).

[136] G. Wu, M. Truksa, N. Datla, P.Vrinten and J. Bauer, *Nature Biotechnology* 23, 1013 (2005).

[137] N. Ruiz-Lopez, R. Haslam, M. Venegas-Caleron, T. Li and J. Bauer, *Transgenic Res.* 8, 1 (2012).

[138] N. Ruiz-Lopez, R.P. Haslam, S.L. Usher, J.A. Napier and O. Sayanova, *Metabolic Engineering* 17, 30 (2013).

[139] J.R. Petrie, P. Shrestha, X.R Zhou, M.P. Mansour and Q. Liu, *PLOS One* 7: e49165 (2012).

[140] J.R. Petrie and S.P Singh, *AOB Plants* doi: 10.1093/aobpla/plr011 (2011).

[141] N Ruiz-Lopez, O. Sayanova, J.A. Napier and R.P. Haslam, *J. Experimental Botany* 63, 2397 (2012).

[142] J.R. Petrie, P. Shrestha, S. Belide, Y. Kennedy and G. Lester, *PLoS ONE* 9, e85061 (2014).

[143] J.R. Petrie, P. Shrestha, X.R. Zhou, M.P. Mansour, Q. Liu, S. Belide, P.D. Nichols and S.P. Singh, *PLoS ONE* 7, e49165 (2012).

[144] N. Ruiz-Lopez, R.P. Haslam, J.A. Napier and O. Sayanova, *The Plant Journal,* 77, 198 (2014).

[145] Knapton, Sarah 2014. GM crops given green light by government at http://www.telegraph.co.uk/science/science-news/10769797/GM-crops-given-green-light-by-government.html

[146] J.A. Hirt-Chabbert, *Adding value to New Zealand eels by aquaculture.* PhD thesis Auckland University of Technology, New Zealand (2011).

In: Marine Oils (From Sea to Pharmaceuticals) ISBN: 978-1-63463-747-3
Editor: Ioannis Zabetakis

Chapter 2

FISH LIPID NUTRITION AND MARINE OILS: FISH REQUIREMENTS OF LIPIDS

Jana Pickova[1,2] and Sofia Trattner[1]
[1]Department of Food Science, Swedish University of Agricultural Sciences, Uppsala, Sweden
[2]University of South Bohemia in České Budějovice, Faculty of Fisheries and Protection of Waters, Research Institute of Fish Culture and Hydrobiology, Vodňany, Czech Republic

ABSTRACT

The presence of fatty acids of aquatic origin is presented in this chapter. Marine oils in fish feeds and thereby the different species requirements are discussed. Focus on larval stages has been chosen as these are not often discussed in connection to fish lipid nutrition and marine oils. Contrary to adult stages, larval fish have very specific needs and parts of larval requirements are still poorly known and understood.

INTRODUCTION

Strong consumer demand for carnivorous fish and shrimp continue to maintain fish oil prices, an ingredient essential for the health and growth of these high-value farmed species. Although human consumption of fish oil is small by comparison with aquaculture utilization, future growth in direct human consumption of fish oils will contribute to upward pressure on fish oil prices. In addition, the production on the global market has decreased caused by lowered catches both in Northern and Southern hemisphere during recent decades as shown on www. thefishsite.com [1]. Peruvian anchovy strongly dominates world fish oil production [2]. It is well established that fish oils are highly regarded for their high proportions of n-3 highly unsaturated fatty acids (HUFA; 20 or more carbons and three or more double bonds),) and taking anchovy oil for example, 20:5n-3 and 22:6n-3 account for about 22% and 9% in total fatty acid (FA), respectively [3]. The proportion between these two fatty acids is greatly more valuable compared to the Northern hemisphere oils.

Fish oil and fish meal have traditionally been and still are used as ingredients in aquafeeds in carnivorous and lately also omnivorous fish species culture. Fish oil has a high level of the n-3HUFA; especially eicosapentaenoic (EPA; 20:5n-3), docosapentaenoic (DPA; 22:5n-3) and docosahexaenoic acid (DHA; 22:6n-3). Fish meal has relatively stable lipid content (8-9%) and the percentage of EPA, DPA and DHA is often higher compared to fish oil. Lately krill (*Euphausia superba*) has become a weighty source of HUFA. Ackman [4] described contents of these fatty acids in fish oils from Northern and Southern hemisphere, respectively, to be different with regards to HUFA. Southern hemisphere oils being richer in EPA and DHA while parts of these FA are replaced by monounsaturated FA in the Northern hemisphere oils. In an investigation by Ahmed et al. [5] of fatty acid composition of fish oil capsules of many brands for human use, purchased in pharmacies and health shops, it could be clearly recognised if the oil originated from menhaden (Southern hemisphere origin) or northern herring oils. Vegetable oils can replace a substantial amount of fish oil in the diets of many fish species without affecting growth and feed conversion efficiency. However, the drawback of these alternatives is the lack of n-3 HUFA, which compromises the nutritive value for different fish species especially for their larval stages and broodstock nutrition. In addition, the value of these fish for human consumption by the amount of HUFA as a specific nutritional component will get hampered.

The requirements of marine oils in total tonnage is clearly most important in the case of ongrowing fish, caused by the excessive feed consumption, but larvae are of importance in this connection as the demands are more absolute and HUFA cannot be replaced by other fatty acids (see below) which has been excellently reviewed by Hamre et al., recently [6].

We know that many different environmental causes have a severe impact on the metabolism of lipids and especially fatty acids in fish. The outer environmental properties such as temperature, light, salinity, predator-prey interactions in wild, feed composition and other cannot be forgotten and all these factors influence the lipid content and composition by altering the metabolism of lipids either in anabolic or catabolic processes. In addition, the fish species and the stage of its life cycle, gender and size are of largest importance as well as the seasonal variations. Many of these factors are still not studied to give enough information of their importance. Especially the larval stages of marine fish species with small eggs require some extra attention as the losses in early stages are costly due to the large demand on egg volume and thereby number of broodstock fish.

DIETARY LIPID REQUIREMENTS

Lipid Classes

Larvae

Larval lipid nutrition has recently been reviewed [6]. Larvae natural conditions are very complex, not only depending on different species, and our knowledge is still based on trials from limited laboratory culture experiments. This lack of knowledge causes mismatch and problems in the early larval stages in culture. Frequent research on lipid requirements in fish larvae, including both essential fatty acids and the ratio of phospholipids (PL) to neutral lipids (NL) has been performed. However, studies aimed at determining the quantitative requirements for these nutrients with dose-response, including at least five dietary levels, are very scarce [6]. Fish larvae fed formulated diets where the lipid is added solely as oils, triacylglycerol (TAG), show often poor growth and survival and show lipid droplets in intestinal tissue and liver. Dietary PL has been found to be required for the growth and survival of a range of species since the early 1980s [7]. Phospholipids are available in high proportion in pelagic fish and crustacean eggs as well as in plankton crustaceans. The fat content of the stages of copepods that are eaten by marine fish larvae, for example juvenile stages, e.g. nauplii and copepodites, is 6–16% of dry matter (DM), where ca 50% of the lipid as PL, depending on stage [8]. Phospholipids are also involved in the digestion, absorption and transport of lipids from the intestine to the larval body. The larvae lack the ability to synthesize PL efficiently to cover their demands and therefore PL need to be included in the diet [7]. The intestine of first feeding larvae is poorly developed and PL synthesis occurs there in fish

[9, 10]. Few studies have shown that PL synthesis occurs mainly through the glycerol-3-phosphate pathway, whose activity is modulated through dietary lipids. As a result of this finding, addition of lecithin into larval microdiets has resulted in improved transport and utilization of dietary lipids and promoting growth [11]. Phospholipid requirements have been found to be related to the larval age and the degree of digestive system development [12]. Several authors have found (see below) that gilthead sea bream (*Sparus aurata*) suffers of growth depression related to insufficient PL contents of the diet. In addition to the PL importance for growth and lipid utilization, dietary PL improves stress resistance, skeleton development and flatfish metamorphosis and pigmentation [6]. PL constitute a wide group of compounds formed by different bases and types of fatty acids, their effect in the larvae may depend on the particular components of the dietary PL source used. Enhanced lipoprotein synthesis can be responsible for the growth promotion effect of phosphatidylcholine, PC, by increasing energy flux from the intestinal mucosa into the blood [13]. PC seems to promote growth better than other PL classes of several species [14, 15] and in addition enhances feeding [16]. Also the type of fatty acids binding to the PL, can vary depending on source, which is of importance since marine fish larvae natural preys such as copepods have a high content of PLs rich in n-3 highly unsaturated fatty acids. One such case is described in larval ayu (*Plecoglossus altivelis*) PL from bonito eggs rich in n-3 highly unsaturated fatty acids improve growth and survival more effectively than PL from a vegetable source. A possible explanation of the results is the different content of essential fatty acids. It has been found that the diet with the highest dietary PL gave the best larval performance and lower skeletal malformation rates for pikeperch (*Sander lucioperca*) larvae [17]. They also showed the best growth with the diet highest in PL (90 g kg-1 DM). In common carp larvae (*Cyprinus carpio*), the opposite was found, an excess of dietary PC was found to decrease survival and to increase the malformation rate [14].

Later Stages

Later stages of many fish species have not specifically been investigated and very little evidence on PL requirement in adult fish is present to date.

Based on studies comparing a neutral lipid-rich commercial diet and a phospholipid-rich zooplankton diet, Olsen et al. [18] suggested that polar lipids may promote growth in juvenile Atlantic cod, but more work is needed to decide on requirements in this and other species. It is suggested that cod larvae and small juveniles may have low digestibility of neutral lipid classes due to a lack of suitable lipases, bile acids or both. During larval and early juvenile periods cod may have an absolute need for polar lipids including PL both for the supply of energy and for essential fatty acids.

However, Atlantic salmon (*Salmo salar*) have several adaptations to digest diets rich in wax esters. This includes increased feed conversion, higher production of bile and higher activity of lipolytic enzymes in the midgut. Atlantic salmon has been shown to feed and grow on diets with a medium amount of wax esters (30% of the lipid) with results comparable to fish maintained on fish oil diets. Ingestion of higher level of wax esters (50% of the lipid) cause, however, poorer lipid digestibility and growth, so that optimal utilization of wax esters in Atlantic salmon is closer to 30% than 50% of the dietary lipid.

In a digestibility study, apparent digestibility coefficients (ADC) of dry matter, lipid and individual fatty acids were always highest in fish fed soybean lecithin diet. In hindgut ADC of lipid and dry matter were 94 and 96%, respectively, in fish fed the soybean lecithin diet compared to 85 and 94% in fish fed linseed oil. There were major ultrastructural differences in the enterocytes, when Arctic char (*Salvelinus alpinus*) was fed the linseed oil diet [18], with substantial accumulations of lipid droplets. This accumulation was not observed in fish fed the lecithin diet. It is suggested that endogenous PL synthesis is insufficient to maintain lipoprotein synthesis in Arctic char when fed diets containing high levels of polyunsaturated fatty acid of total lipid, and that PL should be added to the diets. As mentioned previously, few studies have been conducted but a requirement for PL has not been conclusively demonstrated in adults of any fish species. For example, the trial on cod (Gadus morhua) [19] did not find convincing PL requirement. On the other hand, if fish meal is included in feed formulations, this problem should be avoided.

REQUIREMENTS FOR POLYUNASATURATED FATTY ACIDS

Larvae

There are numerous studies on the effects of essential fatty acids on growth, survival, behaviour and biological functions and processes in marine fish larvae. Similarly to the situation in lipid requirement, very few studies quantify the needs of larvae of the different species. The importance of each fatty acid differs among the different species and in different environments.

Dietary n-3 highly unsaturated fatty acids (HUFA) in feeds both life and formulated such as rotifers, Artemia or microdiets affect larval survival rate and / or growth, as has been found in numerous marine species including turbot (Psetta maxima), sea breams and also in flatfish pigmentation as shown in Rainuzzo et al. and Hamre & Harboe 2008, [20] [21]. Specific studies aimed at determining the quantitative essential fatty acid requirements for marine fish larvae are scarce. A trial enriching rotifers with different levels of n-3 HUFA to determine the essential fatty acid requirements of red sea bream has been conducted [22]; where levels of n-3 HUFA were 4.7–19.7% of total fatty acids (TFA). It was found that the best growth, survival and resistance to stress were obtained with a level of n-3 HUFA of 15% TFA (3.5% n-3 HUFA DM) [22]. When larvae were fed Artemia (n-3 HUFA 4.2–21.0% TFA, total lipids 129–224 g kg-11 DM) the best growth, survival and resistance to stress were obtained with a level of n-3 HUFA of 15.9% TFA (3.8% n-3 HUFA DM, [22]. A study, enriching rotifers with either DHA or EPA, found that both fatty acids significantly improved survival, but only DHA promoted a significantly higher growth [23]. Studies on gilthead sea bream fed four different levels of n-3 HUFA either in rotifers or in microdiets demonstrated that with adequate DHA/EPA ratios (>1.3) the n-3 HUFA requirements for this species are 1.5–2% DM [24, 25]. The n-6 arachidonic acid (ARA) requirements were also determined for gilthead seabream feeding 17 days post hatch larvae in two trials with seven different diets containing graded levels of ARA, but constant n-3 HUFA and DHA/EPA ratios [26]. Atalah et al. [27] [28] confirmed with five different levels of ARA and EPA this ARA requirement for gilthead seabream, and seabass (Dicentrarchus labrax) and recommended an EPA /ARA ratio of 4. Typically a dietary DHA/EPA ratio of 2:1 is found in marine species and thus, it has been suggested as adequate for larval nutrition [7].

A deficiency of n-3 HUFA and high levels (see below) of arachidonic acid (ARA, 20:4 n-6) cause pigmentation disorders in flatfish [7]; these results have been confirmed in other studies [29, 30]. The data indicate that eicosanoids are involved in the development of pigmentation in flatfish, since increasing ARA, which is the precursor of eicosanoids of the 2-series, gives a reduced rate of normal pigmentation after metamorphosis [31]. In addition, McEvoy et al. [31] showed that dietary ARA and eicosapentaenoic acid (EPA, 20:5 n-3) had opposite effects on pigmentation in turbot and Atlantic halibut (Hippoglossus hippoglossus) and found that a brain EPA:ARA ratio of 4:1 gave the best ratio of normal pigmentation while a ratio of <1:1 would give 100% malpigmentation. The EPA: ARA ratios giving different pigmentation rates in the study of Villalta et al. [32] did not affect the growth and survival of the larvae, while the whole body DHA needed for good survival of Atlantic halibut larvae appeared to be only 6.6–6.8% of TFA (dietary level 7.8% of TFA, dietary FAME 140 mg g-1 DM [33], these figures are much lower than that needed for normal pigmentation. Pickova et al. [34], could see effects of EPA /AA /DHA on cod (Gadus morhua) larvae hatching and survival success. It was observed that the higher the level of ARA and the lower the level of n-3 HUFA, the better the survival.

Later Stages

The environmental effects, such as salinity, temperature are interfering with FA requirements and have surely importance for the needs of essential fatty acids. In culture conditions, the green water use, i.e. addition of algae in the culture environment, intensiveness of the culture system should be considered in dose–response studies. In the range of physiological effects of the different fatty acids, requirements should be determined not only in relation to growth and survival, but also to development of other properties of nervous, skeleton and muscle systems [6] of fish.

All fish species are dependent on dietary essential fatty acids 18:2n-6 and 18:3n-3, in line with the requirements of mammals. To what degree the fish after puberty can utilize these two EFA and synthesize fatty acids longer and with more double bonds (HUFA) is very different depending on the species and their life stage, as demonstrated in Atlantic salmon [35]. The time for restoring these fatty acids is dependent on inclusion level, growth rate and the species. Predictions of the effects can be made by using modeling [36, 37]. A recent study on common carp has shown the same pattern of fatty acid related to inclusion [38]. The declining fish populations of many predatory species lead to a higher and higher degree of replacement by farmed fish, which makes aquaculture as the main demand area for the fish oil worldwide. Predatory fish have much higher demands for lipids and proteins compared to fish in other trophic levels, which possess higher ability to metabolise carbohydrates, and feed formulas can contain approx. 30 % carbohydrates while predatory fish formulas contain max 10% carbohydrates. In a study on Atlantic salmon, it was concluded that marine n-3 fatty acids were not net produced when salmon was fed 80% vegetable oil [39]. This leads to the conclusion that higher levels than 20% of EPA and DHA containing oils are essential for the species. There is no absolute requirement known for Atlantic salmon so far. The studies by Ruyter et al. [40] include evidence on the need of EPA and DHA in salmon of

<100g kept in freshwater. Increasing level of ALA, up to 1%, gave faster growth, and an increased level of EPA and DHA made fish perform even better in terms of lower mortality, better growth rate and better feed conversion. On the other hand, LA gave highest mortality and lowest growth rate. Absolute numbers for requirements are to the best of our knowledge still missing in large Atlantic salmon in seawater.

Lipid Metabolism in Fish

Lipids have structural functions in cell membranes, are precursors for eicosanoids, act as carriers for lipid-soluble substances, and are used for energy production. They can be divided into two main classes; neutral lipids and polar lipids. Neutral lipids serve mainly as an energy source and include triacyl-, diacyl- and monoacylglycerols, sterols, sterol esters, free fatty acids and wax esters. Polar lipids are mostly cell membrane constituents and include glycerophospholipids, glyceroglycolipids and sphingolipids [41, 42].

Lipids may be used for energy, incorporation in membranes as phospholipids or storage as reserve lipid in the tissue. When lipids are ingested, an extracellular hydrolysis of lipids by lipase and colipase occurs in stomach, intestine and cecal lumen, with pyloric ceca and anterior intestine being the most important locations. Fatty acids shorter than C10 and glycerol are absorbed through the brush border of the enterocytes. Fatty acids longer than C12 are cleaved and emulsified by bile salts, to form micelles (negatively charged aggregates). These are transported from lumen to brush border and dissociated to fatty acid and diffused across the epithelial membrane [43]. Inside the enterocyte the fatty acids are re-esterified and grouped with proteins to form chylomicra. From the enterocytes, lipids are transported as chylomicra and partly as VLDL though the hepatic portal vein to the liver, where they are further metabolized or directly transported to other tissues through the dorsal aorta as VLDL. It is unclear if fish have a lymphatic system similar to that in mammals. The majority of uptake of lipids and other lipidic compounds is predominantly mediated by lipoproteins while HDL is the main lipoprotein in salmonids [44]. In fish, similarly to mammals, the TAG are removed from the lipoproteins by lipoprotein lipase (LPL) and the liver takes up the remnant as chylomicron [45].

Lipids are suggested by Van Nieuwenhoven [46] to have two possible ways of transport from extra cellular to intra cellular space, either by diffusion or a protein mediated transport, requiring a membrane-bound fatty acid translocase or a fatty acid transport protein (FATP). Intracellular fatty acid binding protein (FABP) transport long chain fatty acids and other hydrophobic compounds. FABP has been reported in salmon muscle and in intestine of fish [47]. The pathways for PL and TAG biosynthesis are generally the same in fish as in mammals. It occurs in the endoplasmatic reticulum. TAG may be stored as lipid droplets in the cytosol or secreted in plasma as VLDL (e.g. hepatocytes).

The polyunsaturated fatty acids 18:2n-6 and 18:3n-3 are considered essential fatty acids in all vertebrate species, although it has been debated whether long chain n-3 fatty acids are essential for marine fish species [48]. In salmonids, it has been shown that the length and degree of unsaturation of the fatty acids decide their metabolic fate [49, 50].

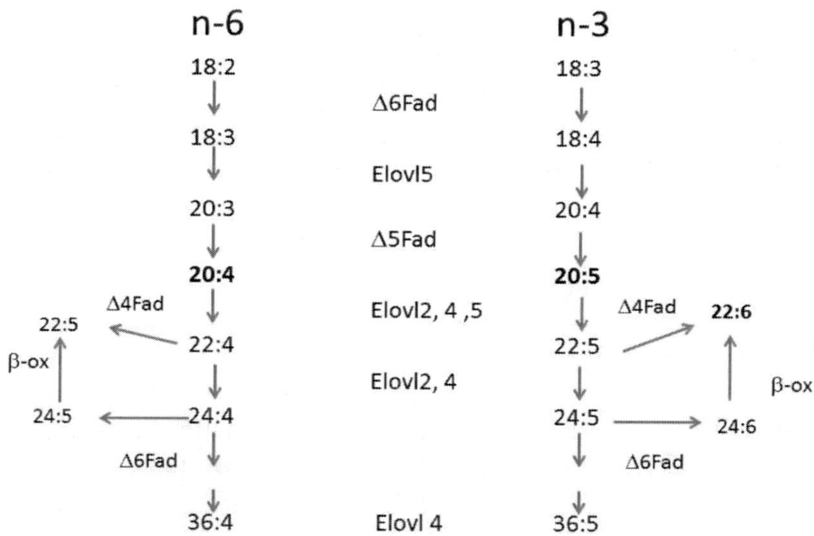

Figure 1. Schematic presentation of possible HUFA pathways in fish FA biosynthesis, adapted rom Voss et al. [56], Navarro-Guillén et al. [52].

Elongation and Desaturation

The biosynthesis pathway from C_{18} to C_{20} and C_{22} is well described for many fresh water species, including rainbow trout (*Oncorhynchus mykiss)* and salmon [42, 50, 51]. Essential substrates for the elongation and desaturation on n-6 and n-3 fatty acids are the 18:2n-6 and 18:3n-3 for all higher vertebrates. The same enzymes are required for both n-6 and n-3 fatty acids, but the affinity of the enzymes are higher for fatty acids of the n-3 series. This synthesis of long chain polyunsaturated fatty acids is occurring in the microsomal fraction of the liver, except the chain shortening reaction to form 22:6n-3, which occurs in peroxisomes. However, the conversion is poorly understood or if at all present in marine species. It has been suggested that the mechanism has been repressed in fish, which has an adequate supply of n-3 HUFA in the natural diet. Recently, results on different pathways in fish of different species have been described [52]. The suggested pathways are presented in Figure 1. Also an elongation to 20:3n-3 exists when 18:3n-3 is present in adequate amount as recently shown in Atlantic salmon [53].

Lipid Catabolism

Red muscle, heart and liver are generally considered as the most important tissues in lipid catabolism [41]. When stored, lipids are catabolised through β-oxidation either heat or ATP will be produced. Heat is produced by the peroxisomal β-oxidation, whereas ATP is produced by mitochondrial β-oxidation. In order to be oxidized, a fatty acid needs to be activated to acyl CoA, which is converted to acylcarnitine by the enzyme carnitine palmitoyltransferase I, to be able to pass the mitochondria inner membrane. Inside the membrane the acylcarnitine will be converted to acyl-CoA by the enzyme carnitine palmitoyltransferase II. The β-oxidation in peroxisomes is mostly oxidizing long chain fatty acids, which can then be further oxidized in the mitochondria or as a step in the synthesis of DHA. Fatty acids have been shown to be selectively β-oxidized with saturated fatty acids as preferred substrate [49]. The main product of peroxisomal β-oxidation in rat hepatocytes is acetate [54]; whereas oxaloacetate and malate originate from mitochondrial β-oxidation. The total β-oxidation is highest in the red muscle followed by the liver and the lowest activity is found in white muscle. Of these tissues, white muscle has the largest proportion of peroxisomal β-oxidation. However in fish having a large proportion of white muscle, a large part of the total β-oxidation will still occur in the white muscle [55].

REFERENCES

[1] (http://www.thefishsite.com/reports/?id=2359#sthash.6Qn6kUVC.dpuf). Accessed 14.02.2014.

[2] S. De Silva, D.S., Francis and A.G.J. Tacon, *Fish Oils in Aquaculture In Retrospect*, in: Turchini, G.M., Ng, W.K., Tocher, D.R. (Eds.) Taylor & Francis (2010).

[3] G.G. Haraldsson and B. Hjaltason In: F.D. Gunstone, (Ed.), *Structured and modified lipids.* Marcel Dekker, New York, pp. 313-350. (2001)

[4] R.G. Ackman Fish oils. In: F. Shahidi, editor. *Bailey´s Industrial oil and fat products,* 6 ed. pp 279–317. (2005)

[5] M.Ahmed, A. Moazzami, R. Andersson, and J.Pickova. *Neuroendocrinology Letters* 32 (SUPPL. 2), pp. 37-40 (2011).

[6] K. Hamre, M. Yufera, I. Rønnestad, C. Boglione, L. E. C. Conceicao and M. Izquierdo. *Reviews in aquaculture* 5 (Suppl. 1), S26–S58 doi: 10.1111/j.1753-5131.2012.01086.x (2013).

[7] J.R. Sargent, L.A. McEvoy and J.G. *Bell Aquaculture* 155: 117–127. (1997)

[8] T. van der Meeren, R.E. Olsen, K. Hamre and H.J. Fyhn. *Aquaculture* 274: 375–397. (2008)

[9] M.F. Sire,C. Lutton, J.M.Vernier. *Journal of Lipid Research* 22: 81–94. (1981).

[10] M.J. Caballero, B.E. Torstensen, L. Robaina, D. Montero and M. Izquierdo. *British Journal of Nutrition* 96: 830–839. (2006b)

[11] J. Liu, M.J. Caballero, M. Izquierdo, T.E.S. Ali, C.M. Hernandez-Cruz, A.Valencia et al. *Fisheries Science* 68: 1165–1172. (2002).

[12] A. Kanazawa. *Journal of the World Aquaculture Society* 24: 162–166. (1993)

[13] I. Seiliez, J.S. Bruant, J.L. Zambonino-Infante, S. Kaushik and P. Bergot *Aquaculture Nutrition* 12: 372–378. (2006)

[14] I. Geurden, O.S. Reyes, P. Bergot, P. Coutteau and P. Sorgeloos. *Fish Physiology and Biochemistry* 19: 365–375. (1998)

[15] E. Hadas, W. Koven, D. Sklan, and A.Tandler. *Aquaculture* 217: 577–588. (2003)

[16] W.M. Koven, G. Parra, S. Kolkovski and A. Tandler. *Aquaculture Nutrition* 4: 39–45. (1998)

[17] N. Hamza, M. Mhetli, I. Ben Khemis, C. Cahu and P. Kestemont. *Aquaculture* 275: 274–282. (2008)

[18] R.E. Olsen. *Journal of Experimental Marine Biology and Ecology* 148: 59-76. (1991)

[19] R.E. Olsen, R. Myklebust,_T. Kaino and E. Ringø_ *Fish Physiology and* Biochemistry 21, 35-44. (1999).

[20] J.R. Rainuzzo, K.I. Reitan Y. Olsen. *Aquaculture* 155: 103–115. (1997)

[21] K. Hamre, A. Srivastava, I. Rønnestad, A. Mangor-Jensen and J. Stoss. *Aquaculture Nutrition* 14: 51–60. (2008b)

[22] M.S. Izquierdo, T. Watanabe, T. Takeuchi, T. Arakawa and C. Kitajima. *Nippon Suisan Gakkaishi* 55: 859–867. (1989)

[23] T. Watanabe T, M.S. Izquierdo, T. Takeuchi, S. Satoh and C. Kitajima. *Nippon Suisan Gakkaishi* 55: 1635–1640. (1989)

[24] C. Rodríguez, J.A. Perez, P. Badia, M.S. Izquierdo, H. Fernandez-Palacios and A.L. Hernández. *Aquaculture* 169: 9–23. (1998)

[25] M. Salhi, M.S. Izquierdo, C.M. Hernández -Cruz, J. Socorro and H. Fernández-Palacios. *Journal of Fish Biology* 51: 869–879. (1997)

[26] M. Bessonart, M.S. Izquierdo, M. Salhi, C.M. Hernández-Cruz, M.M. González and H. Fernández-Palacios. *Aquaculture* 179: 265–275. (1999)

[27] E. Atalah, C.M. Hernández-Cruz, T. Benı´tez-Santana, R. Ganga, J. Roo and M. Izquierdo. *Aquaculture Research* 42: 1279–1288. (2011a)

[28] E. Atalah, C.M. Hernández-Cruz, E. Ganuza, T. Benı´tez-Santana, R. Ganga, J. Roo, et al. *Aquaculture Research* 42: 1261–1268. (2011b)

[29] R.J. Shields, J.G. Bell, F.S. Luizi, B. Gara, N.R. Bromage and J.R. Sargent. *Journal of Nutrition* 129: 1186–1194. (1999)

[30] K. Hamre, E. Holen, M. Moren. *Aquaculture Nutrition* 13: 65–80. (2007)

[31] L.A. McEvoy, A. Estévez, J.G. Bell, R.J. Shields, B. Gara and J.R. Sargent. *Bulletin of the Aquaculture Association of Canada* 98, 4: 17–20. (1998)

[32] M. Villalta, A. Estévez and M.P. Bransden. Aquaculture 245: 193–209. (2005a).

[33] K. Hamre and T. Harboe. Aquaculture 277: 101–108. (2008b).

[34] J. Pickova, P.C. Dutta, P-O. Larsson and A. Kiessling. *Canadian Journal of Fisheries and Aquatic Sciences* 54: 2410-2416. (1997).

[35] J.G. Bell, D.R. Tocher, B.M. Farndale, D.I. Cox, R.W. McKinney, and J.R. Sargent. *Lipids* 32(5), 515-525. (1997).

[36] M. Jobling. *Aquaculture Research* 35:7, 706-709. (2004).

[37] J.H., Robin, C., Regost, J. Arzel, and S.J. Kaushik. *Aquaculture* 225(1-4), 283-293. (2003).

[38] J. Mráz, T.Zajic and J. Pickova. *Neuroendocrinology Letters* 33, Suppl. 2: 60-67. (2012)

[39] N.S. Liland, G. Rosenlund, M.H.G. Berntssen, T. Brattelid, L. and B.E.Torstensen, *Aquaculture Nutrition* 19: 289-300. (2013)

[40] B. Ruyter, C. Røsjø, O. Einen and M.S. Thomassen, *Aquaculture Nutrition 6*: 109-117. (2000)

[41] R.J. Henderson and D.R. Tocher. *Prog. Lipid Res.* 26: 281-347.(1987).

[42] D.R. Tocher, *Reviews in Fisheries Science* 11(2): 107-184. (2003).

[43] E.J., Kleveland, B.L. Syvertsen, B. Ruyter, A. Vegusdal, S.M.Jorgensen and T. Gjøen, *Lipids* 41(11), 1017-1027. (2006b).

[44] P.J. Babin and J-M. Vernier J. *Lipid Res.* 30: 467-489. (1989).

[45] B. Torstensen and D.R. Tocher in Fish oil replacement and alternative lipid sources in Aquaculture feeds, Eds G.M. Turchini, W.K. Ng and D.R. Tocher, CRC Press. 2011. pp 405-438. (2011).

[46] F.A.Van Nieuwenhoven, G.J. VanderVusseand and J.F.C. Glatz. *Lipids* 31,S223-S227. (S Suppl), (1996).

[47] A. Vegusdal, T. Gjøen, R.K Berge, M.S. Thomassen and B. Ruyter. *Lipids* 40 (5):477-486 (2005).

[48] J.R. Sargent, J.G. Bell, M.V. Bell, R.J. Hendersson & D.R. Tocher (1995 *Journal of applied Ichthyology* 11(3-4), 183-198.

[49] K.H. Kiessling and A. Kiessling. *Canadian Journal of Zoology* 71(2): 248-251. (1993).

[50] J.G. Bell, D.R. Tocher, B.M. Farndale, D.I. Cox, R.W. McKinney and J.R. Sargent. *Lipids* 32(5): 515-525. (1997).

[51] M. Buzzi, R.J. Henderson and J.R. Sargent, *Comparative Biochemistry and Physiology B-Biochemistry & Molecular Biology* 116(2), 263-267. (1997).

[52] C. Navarro-Guillén, S. Engrola,F. Castanheira, N. Bandarra, I.Hachero-Cruzado, D. R. Tocher, L.E.C. Conceição and S. Morais (2014) Comparative Biochemistry and Physiology, Part B 167 : 51–58.

[53] J.A. Emery, R.P. Smullen, and G.M. Turchini, 2014. *Aquaculture* 422-423, pp. 98-108.

[54] F. Leighton, S. Bergseth, T. Rortveit, E.N. Christiansen and J. Bremerll, *The Journal of Biological Chemistry* 264, 10347-10350. (1989).

[55] L. Froyland, O. Lie, and R.K. Berge. *Aquaculture Nutrition* 6(2), 85-89. (2000).

[56] A. Voss, M. Reinhart, S. Sankarappa, and H. Sprecher, *Journal of Biological Chemistry* 266(30): 19995-20000. (1991). http://www.thefishsite.com/reports/?id=2359#sthash.6Qn6kUVC.dpuf.

In: Marine Oils (From Sea to Pharmaceuticals) ISBN: 978-1-63463-747-3
Editor: Ioannis Zabetakis

Chapter 3

AQUACULTURE AND FOOD SECURITY

Mags Crumlish
Institute of Aquaculture, Stirling University, Stirling, Scotland, UK

ABSTRACT

Food security is a complex issue with many external factors influencing our ability to provide safe and nutritious food products for human consumption. There are numerous descriptions applied to what food security means but for the purposes of this chapter we shall explore the nutritional role and value of farmed seafood within global food security. The capture fisheries sector remains relatively static and unlikely to expand further, meaning that more of our edible seafood will be provided from aquatic farming systems. As seafood is one of the most highly traded food commodities worldwide, this suggests that there is a significant role for aquaculture within food security. This chapter will describe the contribution of aquaculture products within global food security and explore the relationship between existing and novel marine oil sources required for sustainable aquaculture production. We will discuss the need for fish/marine oil sources in aquafeeds and the approaches taken by the fish farming industry to include alternative sources and feeding strategies to reduce the pressure on these vital raw marine ingredients within aquafeeds. We shall introduce the malnutrition burden facing our increasing global population impacting on human health and the competition for the marine sources of long chain omega-3 fatty acids (LC omega-3), within the modern agri-food sector.

Aquatic Food Security and Aquaculture

Food security was defined by the World Food Summit in 1996 as "situation that exists when all people at all times, have physical, social and economic access to sufficient, safe and nutritious food that meets their dietary needs and preferences for an active and healthy life". When considering food security we must remember that we no longer live in isolation and many of our dietary staples are intensively farmed and globally transported. Any food production therefore, is influenced by physical access, economic wealth and political stability, at both the national and international level all of which can heavily impact on nutritional equality and human health. According to Friel and Lichacz (2010) [1] we now live in a world with unequal food systems and unhealthy diets, resulting in a double burden of malnutrition affecting the global population. Perhaps we consider malnutrition to equate only to undernutrition or a lack of food but it can now be applied to overnutrition, a consequence of which is the growing obesity epidemic already prevalent in some countries. Malnutrition in the broadest sense will impact on human health and welfare but how this manifests itself will depend on whether it is due to a lack or an abundance of calories in our diets.

The contribution of seafood within food security is not well recognized and yet aquatic food provides more than 3 billion people with approximately 15% of their animal protein intake [2]. As a food type, seafood is extremely diverse, sold both nationally and internationally as whole animals, dressed or undressed fillets as well as in various ready-to-eat formats. All of these products are traded globally with the produce harvested from capture fisheries, aquaculture or a combination of both. The supply of seafood from the capture fisheries sector is in decline [3] and so aquatic farmed products are likely to provide the majority of the seafood sold and consumed on the international market. The actual figures related to decline in the capture fisheries sector is much debated however, the overall trend shows a decline. This may stabilize over time but there will continue to be greater reliance on aquaculture to provide our seafood products suitable for human consumption (Figure 1). Aquatic farming, also called aquaculture is not a new activity but the development and socio-economic benefit from this food sector continues to grow as in 2012, the world aquaculture production was estimated to have reached 66 million tones with a farm-gate value of US$ 138 billion [4]. At present, aquaculture is the fastest growing food production sector with more than 600 food fish and algal species being farmed for human consumption in more than 190 countries worldwide [4].

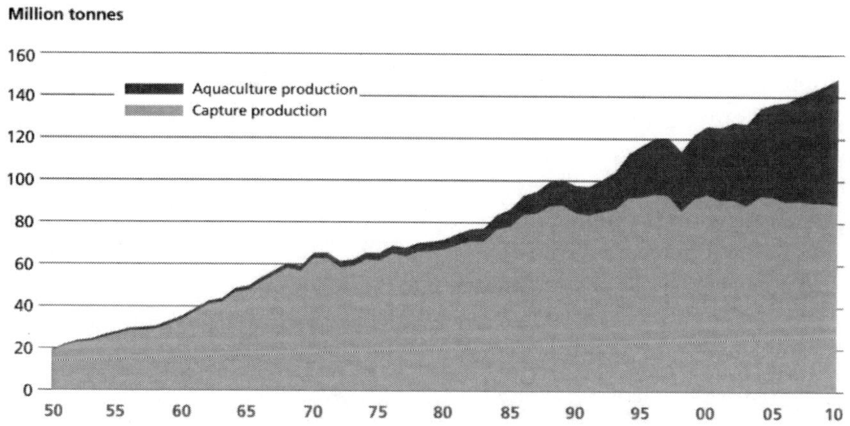

Figure 1. State of the world capture fisheries and aquaculture production reproduced from The State of World Fisheries and Aquaculture, UNFAO (2012) [4].

It is fair to say that there are strengths and weaknesses in all farming sectors but the key assets in aquatic farming include the range of production systems, diversity of aquatic farmed species and the relatively lower production costs compared with our terrestrial farming systems.

The diversity of food produced from our aquatic ecosystems is vast and compared with other farming sectors aquaculture has the more sustainable growth potential therefore the contribution of aquaculture within global food security is only recently being recognized.

Nutritionally, more than 1 billion people rely on fish as the primary animal protein in their diets [3, 4] where the average annual fish consumption is 16.1 kg per capita globally. In terms of human health, fish provide a range of essential vitamins, minerals, protein and oils.

As such, fish or fish products are widely marketed as an important part of a balanced and healthy human diet. There is no doubt that fish provide a nutritionally competent food source and have been described as one of the original “superfoods”.

Although this term is not officially recognized and is not supported in food packaging within the EU (www.nhs.uk) it is widely applied in the general food industry to mean a food source that has added health benefits over and above the actual measurable nutritional value.

These additional benefits often include vitamins and antioxidants or in the case of fish, it is the essential fatty acids. The human body cannot make these essential fatty acids so must acquire them through their diet.

The fatty acids important for human health belong to the long chain omega-3 polyunsaturated fatty acids (LC omega-3 PUFA), particularly eicosapentaenoic acid (EPA) and docosahexaenoic acid (DHA) [5].

Many government bodies and health regulatory departments recommend inclusion of LC omega-3 food sources as part of a healthy and balanced diet. Of course there are numerous dietary sources of these essential fatty acids including terrestrial plants and seeds, but one of the best sources of dietary omega-3 is from farmed salmon.

Most of the salmon sold on the global market are farmed Atlantic salmon (*Salmo salar*) where in Scotland the farmed production has increased from 14 tonnes in 1971 to 162,000 tonnes in 2012 (www.SSPO). This fish is of commercial importance to Norway, Scotland and Chile and it is now considered as Scotland's leading food export (www.SSPO). As with humans, the salmon must acquire the fatty acids from their diet and in the wild this would come from either microalgae which are a natural source of the LC omega-3 or by eating smaller prey fish which has bioaccumulated the fatty acids naturally. Salmon are carnivorous fish and in non-farming conditions would naturally eat smaller fish species providing the dietary fatty acids that the salmon could then use as an energy source for growth and development. Of course we are concerned with farmed fish and in salmon production units worldwide, the animals are feed on commercially manufactured feeds to provide the balanced ingredients required for optimal growth and development. The aquafeed sector has invested in research and development to produce the farmed salmon with a high quality diet optimally balanced with all of the essential ingredients, including fish oil. Unlike other carnivorous species, the salmon accumulate the fish oils within their flesh, making the LC omega-3 easily available when the salmon are consumed.

Aquaculture and Fish Oil

The fishmeal and fish oil included in the salmon diets have traditionally been provided by capture fisheries and included pelagic species often not suited for human consumption directly. Typically these include small boney and oily fish such as anchovy, horse mackerel and pilchard amongst others [6].

These raw marine resources are in finite supply and according to Hardy (2010) [7] if the aquaculture sector continue to demand wild fish as a source of fishmeal and fish oil at higher levels than those naturally available, aquaculture would no longer be a food producer but a direct consumer.

This would increase the already heavy burden placed within food security rather than alleviate some of the pressure. Therefore alternative marine oil sources or feeding strategies for aquaculture must be investigated if it is to have a sustainable future and positive contribution in food security. For the purposes of this chapter we will only consider fish oil.

Although the annual data of fish oil required for aquaculture purposes fluctuates, the overall trend has been a steady increase in demand aligned with the growth of the aquatic farming sector, particularly for marine carnivorous fish. Over the last 20 years the global increase in fish oil being used for aquaculture has increased from 15 to 85% [8]. The persistent demand for marine oil within aquafeeds sourced from a single dietary source (pelagic fish) is not only risky but places an unsustainable pressure on our valuable marine ecosystems. This has been recognized by the aquaculture sector and much progress has been made to identify alternatives to both fishmeal and fish oil for inclusion in the aquafeed sector.

Before we explore the alternative sources we should consider how the essential fatty acids are being applied in human health and how this relates to food security. Inclusion of essential fatty acids in the human diet has been ascribed to numerous health benefits including a measureable reduction or prevention in cardiovascular disease [9]. Clinical trials have also shown that intake of LC omega-3 can reduce blood pressure [10] and may even contribute to improved mental health and alertness [11] for some patients. Deficiencies of LC omega-3 in our diet can lead to developmental abnormalities and can contribute towards many preventable deaths [12]. The mode-of-action of fatty acids is still being clarified but they have been shown to affect the cellular membrane composition, function and cell signaling pathways [12] and so play a crucial role in maintaining a healthy lifestyle. Leaf and Weber [13] (1987) described the dietary changes in our fatty acid intake from nutritional sources over the last 1000 years, from early hunter-gather to farmer and now predominantly consumer. They clearly show the relationship between lifestyle change and food production over time. In our era of modern food production not only has the total amount of dietary fat increased but the ratio of essential fatty acids have changed resulting in lower LC omega-3 and higher omega-6 levels. The modern diet can have a ratio as high as 15:1 for LC omega-6 and omega-3, respectively, where a more beneficial range for human health is 3:1 or 5:1 omega-6 to omega 3, respectively [6]. As oily fish are a unique source of these LC omega-3 fatty acids then consuming 2 portions per week will help to rebalance our dietary intake helping to support our growth and development as well as contribute towards healthy lifestyle choices.

Of course, a quick Internet search shows that we do not need to consume whole fish or fish products to achieve our recommended daily intake of LC omega-3. We can instead purchase supplements or other functional foods that have added or enhanced LC omega-3. This is part of a growing "wellness" trend, particularly prevalent in the western world and driven by the nutraceutical sector [1].

The term functional food first appeared in Japan in the 1980's and has evolved to include *foods that provide health benefits beyond basic nutrition* [14]. The modern food production sector embraces functional food or human wellness as an important part of their future growth and provide substantial resources to the research and development of many function foods. The growth of this agri-food sector provides additional competition for raw marine ingredients high in essential fatty acids.

In many western countries, food and nutrition is a personal choice, not often constrained by lack of access or availability. Of course one could argue that this has contributed towards the obesity epidemic as we consume high levels of nutritionally inadequate food in large portions. It is not our intention to discuss food or diet choices and whilst functional foods or fish oil capsules may provide a proportion of our essential fatty acids, their contribution towards human health and wellness will be limited compared with eating whole fish. This competition for marine ingredients between the nutraceutical and aquaculture sector will only add to global food insecurity and fuel the global malnutrition burden.

Nevertheless, the demand for nutritionally superior food types or dietary supplements continues to grow, particularly in western populations. Ingestion of a daily fish oil capsule may readdress the nutritional imbalance for some individuals, but it is an expensive and long-term investment to acquire essential fatty acids in our diet compared with eating 2 portions of oily fish per week. The daily intake of LC omega-3 is recommended at 0.25g to 0.5g per person per day. Eating 2 portions of fish per week with at least 1 being an oily fish will provide 3g per week of LC omega-3 [6].

Government and health authorities in many countries support this recommendation within a healthy, balanced diet. Furthermore quality control standards are not universally applied within the nutraceutical sector, therefore all supplements or functional foods will not be of equal nutritional benefit. This increased demand for the limited supply of raw marine ingredients will impact heavily on the sustainability of our aquaculture industry and the development of the nutraceutical sector, unless alternative LC omega-3 resources can be identified.

Alternative Dietary Oil Sources for Aquaculture

Alternative sources of LC omega-3 could be provided from non-fish sources including terrestrial plants, animals and marine microalgae. Significant research is required prior to implementing any dietary changes or substitutions within the aquafeeds produced for our farmed fish. Glencross et al. (2010) [15] provide an excellent review on the key considerations required to evaluate ingredients within aquaculture feeds. Of particular importance are the characterization, digestibility, palatability and nutritional uptake and function of the dietary ingredients [15]. The global production from terrestrial farmed grains and oilseeds has increased over the last 20 years and these may provide an alternative source of oil [7] suitable for aquafeeds. Much research has been completed in finding suitable alternative vegetable based fatty acids for inclusion in the farmed fish diets [16, 17]. In terms of the farmed salmon diet it was shown that inclusion of terrestrial-based vegetable oils did not compromise fish growth, health or quality of the animals produced [18, 19] meaning that this is a viable option within aquaculture. It is widely recognized that vegetable-based oils contain lower levels of LC-PUFA resulting in lower levels of essential fatty acids in the fish flesh [20]. This has been shown irrespective of whether the vegetable oils are provided in the fish diet as singularly or as a blended mix. Bell et al. (2004) [19] suggested 50% or less replacement of the fish oil with the vegetable based oil, otherwise there was a significant reduction in the LC omega-3 present in the salmon flesh. This would be an unwelcome outcome in terms of the human health benefits in eating farmed oily fish and lessen the positive contribution of this aquaculture sector within global food security as it would lessen the nutritional value of the fish products consumed.

But perhaps there is another way of including the vegetable oil sources within the aquafeed diet. The aquaculture industry has not excluded the vegetable based oils as replacement sources in the salmon diet, but instead have investigated their inclusion within alternative feed strategies. Bell et al. (2010) [21] showed that the LC omega-3 fatty acid levels could be restored in salmon by including a 16-week fish oil finisher diet, even though the fish had been predominantly fed vegetable oil at 65% replacement during the bulk of the production cycle. In the manufactured feed industry uptake of this approach is increasing thus ensuring a high quality nutritionally valuable fish product that has been raised more sustainably.

Other sources of suitable replacement oils for aquaculture diets have been explored including those from terrestrial animals, microalgae, krill, calamari and genetically modified crops [22]. Whilst they all have their strengths and weaknesses, the most promising alternative may arise from the marine microalgae particularly as they are primary producers of the essential fatty acids rich in EPA and DHA [22]. Microalgae are an established live food resource for filter feeding shellfish and fish larvae in a wide range of aquaculture practices [22] (Table 1). There are several phyla and species of marine microalgae that have shown potential as suitable sources of essential fatty acids, all of which could be sustainably resourced and included in a wide range of aquafeeds. Ryckebosch et al. (2014) [22] showed that microalgae oils sourced from species belonging to *Isochrysis*, *Nannochloropsis*, *Phaeodactylum*, *Pavlova* and *Thalassiosira* all provided sufficient quality and quantity of essential fatty acids to serve as a dietary alternative for fish oil when administered in the farmed fish diet. They even went as far as suggesting that including the microalgae oil as the primary source of essential oils in the fish diet may provide even more human health benefits when fish fed these feed sources are consumed as the microalgae contain additional dietary factors which could accumulate in the fish flesh [21]. Microalgae can be produced in a wide range of habitats, making them a particularly attractive source of LC omega-3 alternatives, as algae production would not necessarily compete with space from terrestrial farming resources that are already under tremendous pressure.

Table 1. Commercial Algal Culture and their Application in Aquaculture

Algae	Application in Aquaculture
Nannochloropsis	Live food source for fish larvae and rotifers as naturally high in polyunsaturated fatty acids.
Pavlova	Nutritional enrichment of rotifers fed to fish larvae to raise levels of LC omega-3 (particularly DHA/EPA) in fish and shellfish broodstock.
Isochrysis	Administered as food source in shellfish and shrimp hatcheries.
Tetraselmis	Included in larval shrimp and shellfish feeds.
Thalassiosira weissflogu	Given to shrimp and shellfish hatcheries and useful for shellfish brood stock.
Dunaliella	Used to raise vitamin levels in shrimp hatchery
Chaetoceros	Used to raise vitamin levels in shrimp hatchery

Resourced from [22].

Microalgae are currently used in aquaculture as live feed for a range of commercially important molluscs, crustaceans and fish [23]. However, in the context of this chapter we shall consider them as alternative sources of the LC omega-3 oils added to fish diets. For them to be serious contenders as alternative LC omega-3 sources for aquafeeds significant investment is required to improve commercial production of the microalgae. At present relatively small volumes of the algae are produced and commercially harvested. Significant financial investment is required before this production sector could be scaled–up to meet the persistent demand required for their inclusion in either salmon aquafeeds or nutraceutical supplements. Over the last 50 years commercial microalgae research has explored their potential as alternative sources for a wide range of biochemical products, but this research and development has mostly been led by the biofuel sector [24]. It has been shown that various high value chemical compounds may be extracted from many microalgae including pigments, antioxidants, and vitamins as well as essential fatty acids. The type of product produced depends on the algal species [22].

Production of the microalgae for these biologically active substances requires controlled cultivation systems with high production efficiency. Understanding the varied needs of the different microalgae species when produced under commercial culture conditions can certainly improve the production of essential fatty acids [25]. Large-scale culture of the most beneficial algae will improve with advances in biotechnology but already studies have shown that the influence of the growth conditions is important for the nutritional competency of the algae as a food substitution. As a substitute in aquafeeds it is the delivery of various LC omega-3 fatty acids extracted from the microalgae that will be particularly valuable. Guedes et al. (2010) [26] showed that changes in light intensity altered the lipid profile of the algae *Pavlova lutheri* where lower light intensities provided higher fractions of EPA and DHA.

Total reliance on a single food source to produce a vital dietary ingredient is a risky strategy particularly in a farming sector and this is no different for the aquafeed industry. Spolaore et al. (2006) [27] showed that a combination of different microalgae species provided a better nutritional balance compared with a single species when incorporated into aquafeeds. The ability to extract essential fatty acids from a wide range of microalgae species is certainly an additional benefit in their use as a dietary alternative source of oil for aquafeeds. Nevertheless, any dietary substitutions must be rigorously evaluated for nutritional value and safety in the animals as well as maintaining a high quality food product for human consumption. Therefore if the microalgae are to be suitable replacements in the fish feeds then they need to meet essential criteria similar to other foods sources including low toxicity and high nutritional value.

At present the culture of microalgae has been most successfully applied to aquaculture as a live food source for mollusc, crustacean and fish larvae. For aquatic farmed fish to reach their full potential in resolving some of the dietary imbalances affecting global food security, alternative sources of fish oil are required. Intensive monocultures and commercial harvesting of the microalgae species producing the LC omega-3 oils are not yet fit-for-purpose to supply the high demand as a complete dietary replacements in aquafeeds. However, we have explored some of the available options and how these are currently being addressed. If complete dietary substitution in aquaculture feeds is not possible, perhaps alternative feeding strategies may be a suitable short-term compromise. At present salmon farmers are applying special feeding regimes throughout the production cycle including the use of finishing diets at the latter end of the production cycle to restore the LC omega-3 flesh levels in the salmon. This strategy does not compromise fish growth or development nor the nutritional value of the end-product sold on the international market. It is a sensible approach to using alternative dietary oil ources within aquaculture whilst reducing pressure on the finite marine sources. This approach means that farmed salmon can continue to have a valuable contribution within food security by delivering a more sustainably produced high value product onto the global food market. The financial, environmental and technological challenges of any nutritional changes applied within commercial aquaculture systems must be seriously considered prior to implementation. These challenges are by no mean insurmountable but they must be measured against their contribution within the 3 pillars of food security [28]. This chapter has explored some of the strengths and weaknesses when considering the role of aquatic farmed fish in global food security.

References

[1] S. Friel and W. Lichacz, Unequal Food Systems, Unhealthy Diets In: *Food Security, Nutrition and Sustainability*. Eds. G. Lawrence, K. Lyons and T. Wallington Earthscan ISBN 978-1-84407-775-5 (2010).

[2] M. D. Smith, C. A. Roheim, L. B. Crowder, B. S. Halpern, M. Turnipseed, J. L. Anderson, F. Asche, L. Bourillon, A. G. Guttormsen,

A. Khan, L. A. Liguori, A. McNevin, M. I. O'Connor, D. Squires, P. Tyedmers, C. Brownstein, K. Carden, D. H. Klinger, R. Sagarin, and K. A. Selkoe, *Science* 327, 784 (2010).
[3] J. F. Muir, *Animal Frontiers* 3, 28, (2013).
[4] FAO, The State of the Worlds Fisheries and Aquaculture, Food and Agriculture Organization of the United Nations, Rome (2012) www.fao.org/docrep/016/i2727e.pdf.
[5] G. Ludevese-Pascal, M. D. Pena and J. Tornalejo, *Aquaculture Research* DOI: 10.1111/are.12494 (2014).
[6] H. Pike and A. Jackson, *Lipid Technology* 22, 59 (2010).
[7] R. W. Hardy, *Aquacult. Res.* 41, 770 (2010).
[8] G. J. Tacon and M. Metian, *Aquaculture* 285, 146 (2008).
[9] P. M. Kris-Etherton, W. S. Harris and L. J. Appel, *Circulation* 106, 2747 (2002).
[10] P. R. Howe, *Ann. N Y Acad. Sci.* 827, 339 (1997).
[11] K.-P. Su, S.-Y. Huang, C.-C. Chiu, W. W. Shen, *European Neuropsychopharmacology*, 14, 267 (2003).
[12] G. Danaei, E. L. Ding, D. Mozaffarium, B. Taylor, J. Rehm, C. J. L. Murray, M. Ezzati, *PLoS Med.* 6, 1 (2009).
[13] A. Leaf and P. C. Weber, *Am. J. Clin. Nutr.* 45, 1048-1053 (1987).
[14] C. Hasler, *Food Technology* 52, 63 (1998).
[15] B. D. Glencross, M. Booth and G. L. Allan, *Aquaculture Nutrition* 13, 17 (2010).
[16] S. Hixson, C. C. Parrish, D. M. Anderson, *Food Chemistry* 157, 51 (2014).
[17] G. M. Turchini, B. E. Torstensen, W.-K. Ng, *Rev. Aquaculture* 1, 10 (2009).
[18] J. G. Bell, J. McEvoy, D. R. Tocher, F. McGhee, P. J. Campbell, J. R. Sargent, *J. Nutr.* 131, 1535 (2001).
[19] J. G. Bell, R. J. Henderson, D. R. Tocher, J. R. Sargent, *Lipids* 39, 223 (2004).
[20] B. E. Torstensen, O. Lie, L. Froyland, *Lipids* 35, 653 (2000).
[21] J. G. Bell, J. Pratoomyot, F. Strachan, R. J. Henderson, R. Fontanillas, A. Hebard, D. R. Guy, D. Hunter, D. R. Tocher, *Aquaculture* 306, 225 (2010).
[22] E. Ryckebosch, C. Bruneel, R. Termote-Verhalle, K. Goiris, K. Muylaert, I. Foubert, *Food Chemistry* 160, 393 (2014).
[23] S. Hemaiswarya, R. Raja, R. R. Kumar, V. Ganesan, C. Anbazhagan, *World J. Microbiol. Biotechnol.* 27, 1737 (2011).

[24] T. Mata, A. A. Martins, N. S. Caetano, *Renewable and Sustainable Energy Reviews* 14, 217 (2010).

[25] F. Shahidi, In: *Marine Nutraceuticals and Functional Foods* Eds. C. Barrow and F. Shahidi, Pub. CRC Press ISBN-10: 1574444875 (2007).

[26] C. Guedes and F. X. Malcata, Nutritional Value and Uses of Microalgae in Aquaculture. In: *Aquaculture*, Ed. Dr. Zainal Muchlisin ISBN 978-953-307-974-5, InTech, http://www.intechopen.com/books/aquaculture/nutritional-value-and-uses-of-microalgae-in-aquaculture (2012).

[27] P. Spolaore, C. Joannis-Cassan, E. Duran, A. Isambert, *J. Biosci. Bioeng.* 101, 87 (2006).

[28] World Health Organization (WHO) http://www.who.int.

In: Marine Oils (From Sea to Pharmaceuticals) ISBN: 978-1-63463-747-3
Editor: Ioannis Zabetakis

Chapter 4

MARINE OILS AND DISEASES

Ioannis Zabetakis
Laboratory of Food Chemistry, Faculty of Chemistry, School of Sciences, National and Kapodistrian University of Athens, Athens, Greece

ABSTRACT

The link between marine oils and diseases with particular focus on cardiovascular diseases (CVDs) is presented in this chapter. The scientific evidence that lies behind the justification of the Mediterranean Diet is described in detail. This evidence has given rise to an on growing interest for fish, marine oils and fish oils in our quest to tackle CVDs which is still the number one cause of death in all the countries of the world.

INTRODUCTION

In the history of human's civilisation, people were originally hunters, thus nomadic and their food was dependant on their hunting skills and the availability of animals fit for human consumption. It could be argued that Eurasian civilization is not a product of ingenuity, but of opportunity and necessity. That is, civilization is not created out of superior intelligence, but is the result of a chain of developments, each made possible by certain preconditions.

In our quest to have an insight on the relationship between the consumption of marine oils and the onset of diseases, it would be rather useful to have a retrospective view on how our civilisation has evolved and which forces have been the driving forces over the past millennia.

The first step towards civilization has been the move from nomadic hunter-gatherer to rooted agrarian. Several conditions have been necessary for this transition to occur:

- access to high protein vegetation that endures storage,
- a climate dry enough to allow storage and
- access to animals docile enough for domestication and versatile enough to survive captivity.

Control of crops and livestock has led to the production of food surpluses. These surpluses have freed people to specialize in activities other than maintenance and has supported the growth of population. This combination of specialization and population growth has resulted in the accumulation of social and technologic innovations that have built on each other. Larger societies developed ruling classes and supporting bureaucracies, which in turn led to the organization of nation states and empires. The distribution of wealth and power among societies around the world has been powerfully shaped by biogeographic factors and that environmental endowment has sharply favored some societies, indeed some continents, over others. This has made it highly probable that these "lucky" ones would in time prevail over the "unlucky" [1].

The parts of the world that have been fortunate enough to have a large share of potentially domesticable plants and animals, and located so as to favour the migration and diffusion of domesticated plants and animals, developed farming, metallurgy, writing, states, among others than other societies did. According to Diamond [1], the ultimate cause of success of some civilizations over others was: a favorable environmental endowment.

Nowadays, a similar phenomenon is observed but with somewhat reversed gravity. The westernized societies suffer from Cardiovascular Diseases (CVDs) to a greater population ratio than some not so "developed" societies in terms of GDP or wealth.

However, the projections of death causes for all countries, irrespective of the level of income, suggest that ischaemic heart disease (and thus CVDs) is the primary disease or injury and will still be responsible for the majority of deaths in 2030 [2].

Income Group	Rank	Disease or Injury	Percent of Total Deaths
World	1	Ischaemic heart disease	13.4
	2	Cerebrovascular disease	10.6
	3	HIV/AIDS	8.9
	4	COPD	7.8
	5	Lower respiratory infections	3.5
	6	Trachea, bronchus, lung cancers	3.1
	7	Diabetes mellitus	3.0
	8	Road traffic accidents	2.9
	9	Perinatal conditions	2.2
	10	Stomach cancer	1.9
High-income countries	1	Ischaemic heart disease	15.8
	2	Cerebrovascular disease	9.0
	3	Trachea, bronchus, lung cancers	5.1
	4	Diabetes mellitus	4.8
	5	COPD	4.1
	6	Lower respiratory infections	3.6
	7	Alzheimer and other dementias	3.6
	8	Colon and rectum cancers	3.3
	9	Stomach cancer	1.9
	10	Prostate cancer	1.8
Middle-income countries	1	Cerebrovascular disease	14.4
	2	Ischaemic heart disease	12.7
	3	COPD	12.0
	4	HIV/AIDS	6.2
	5	Trachea, bronchus, lung cancers	4.3
	6	Diabetes mellitus	3.7
	7	Stomach cancer	3.4
	8	Hypertensive heart disease	2.7
	9	Road traffic accidents	2.5
	10	Liver cancer	2.2
Low-income countries	1	Ischaemic heart disease	13.4
	2	HIV/AIDS	13.2
	3	Cerebrovascular disease	8.2
	4	COPD	5.5
	5	Lower respiratory infections	5.1
	6	Perinatal conditions	3.9
	7	Road traffic accidents	3.7
	8	Diarrhoeal diseases	2.3
	9	Diabetes mellitus	2.1
	10	Malaria	1.8

DOI: 10.1371/journal.pmed.0030442.t003

Figure 1. Ten Leading Causes of Death, by Income Group, 2030 (Baseline Scenario) [2].

Cardiovascular Diseases

Today, according to the latest data available, CVDs are the number one cause of death globally: more people die annually from CVDs than from any other cause. An estimated 17.3 million people died from CVDs in 2008 alone, representing 30% of all global deaths [3, 4]. Of these deaths, an estimated 7.3 million were due to coronary heart disease and 6.2 million were due to stroke [4]. Low-income and middle-income countries are disproportionally affected: over 80% of CVD deaths take place in low- and middle-income countries and occur almost equally in men and women [3].

Also, the number of people who die from CVDs, mainly from heart disease and strokes, will increase to reach 23.3. million by 2030 [2, 3].

Thirty years after the study of the 7 countries [5], there are still some questions on why some cohorts had coronary heart disease (CHD) at low frequencies but high levels of serum cholesterol (Figure 2 and 3).

In the following two figures, it can be seen that in westernized societies the higher the serum cholesterol the higher the mortality by CHD. However, in southern Europe and in Japan, this phenomenon is not observed. Since this 7-countries study, life scientists have started looking into the diet that populations in southern Europe and in Japan follow in order to establish whether specific foods could be associated with the onset of CVDs.

MEDITERRANEAN DIET

Today, cardiovascular diseases (CVDs), although preventable, remain the top global cause of death and stroke [7] and our focus (and one of the aims of this book) should be to suggest ways to increase food functionality against CVDs in a sustainable way. One of the major objectives of research in life sciences should be the prevention of CVDs and atherosclerosis and we should study more vigorously how specific food components participate in the atherosclerotic mechanism(s) involved and how we can ensure sustainable production of these components [8].

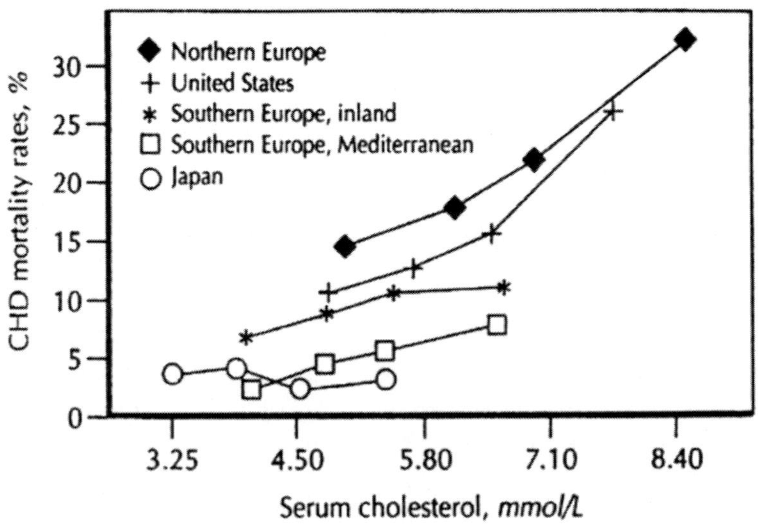

Figure 2. Rate of mortality due to Coronary Heart Disease (CHD) per quartile of serum cholesterol in pooled cohorts of the Seven Countries Study [6].

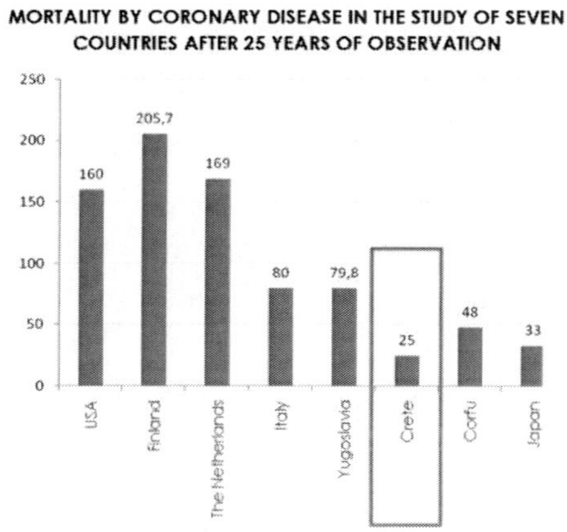

Adapted from [6].

Figure 3. Average mortality per 1000 people (lowest results for Crete and Corfu in Greece and also Japan).

The onset and the development of CVDs are somehow multifactorial phenomena that arise out of an interaction of different combinations of risk factors. Particular combinations can be especially atherogenic, i.e. leading to the onset of atherogenesis in our blood arteries and eventually CVDs.

Risk factors can be categorized as:

- physiological factors (e.g. blood pressure, plasma cholesterol)
- uncontrollable factors (i.e. background factors) (e.g. height, sex, social class, geographical location) and
- controllable factors (i.e. behavioural factors) (e.g. exercise, diet, smoking, stress).

Many of the behavioural factors may exert their effects through a number of different physiological risk factors. Obesity, for example, which is defined as having a Body Mass Index (BMI) higher than 30, in conjunction with excessive central fat deposition could lead to high blood pressure, increased plasma insulin levels and increased plasma cholesterol levels; all these are physiological factors that increase the risk of CVDs.

Sometimes, a behavioural factor can have a beneficial effect on some risk factors, yet it can have a detrimental effect, i.e. increasing risk in others. The consumption of alcohol is a good example.

Heavy and irregular alcohol consumption can increase blood pressure, although regular moderate consumption of alcohol can reduce the build-up of fibrous plaque and thus reduce likelihood of a blood clot (see Figure 4 where moderate wine consumption is suggested!).

The onset of CVDs is atherosclerosis which is defined as a chronic inflammatory condition caused by the deposition of cholesterol and other cellular constituents in the intima of large and medium arteries [10] and it can lead to an acute clinical event through plaque rapture and thrombosis. In atherosclerosis, Platelet Activating Factor (PAF) [11] plays a crucial role [12].

Modern research in life sciences focuses on assessing the biological activities of food components against CVDs and structurally elucidating the food components with such specific cardioprotective properties. This approach should give valuable molecular and biological insights into the role of specific food in preventing atherosclerosis, and thus, providing cardioprotection [13].

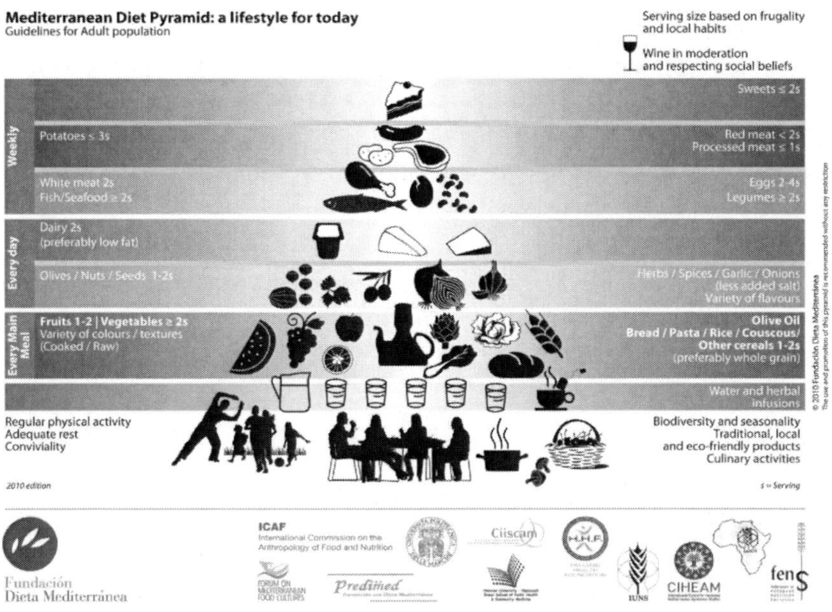

Figure 4. The current Mediterranean diet pyramid that includes guidelines for regular physical activity, culinary activities and consuming food in companion with other people [9].

PHYSIOLOGICAL FUNCTIONS OF MARINE OILS

As mentioned previously in this book, marine oils are excellent sources of fatty acids (FAs), monounsaturated FAs (MUFAs) and polyunsaturated FAs (PUFAs). In humans, FAs, MUFAs and PUFAs play a number of beneficial physiological roles.

Initially, they can all act as a energy source and, in the form of phospholipids, they are the structural components of all cell membranes, affecting the thickness and also the fluidity of the membranes and subsequently the activity of the proteins associated to membranes. They also play an important role as sources of intracellular signals in response to extracellular ones that interact with receptors on the external layer of the plasma membrane [14, 15].

Fatty acids function also as precursors of lipid mediators, with eicosanoids as the most vital ones. Eicosanoids [e.g. prostaglandinds (PG), thromboxanes (TX) and leukotrienes (LT)] act as hormones with an autocrine or paracrine action. Moreover, FAs have a functional role in cell signaling pathways, as ligands of receptors or modulators of gene transcription [16].

The role of marine derived FAs, MUFAs and PUFAs in the onset of various diseases has been extensively studied over the past few decades. Our aim in this book is not to produce a literature review; other colleagues have produced substantial reviews and there is no need to produce one more.

Our aim though is to highlight some strengths and weaknesses of the so far performed studies and suggest constructive ways for future research. Our approach in presenting the studies on the role of marine oils is this: we have divided the studies into:

1 in vitro studies
2 in vivo studies and
3 dietary interventions

and in the following two chapters all these studies are presented and critically evaluated. In chapter 5, the *in vitro* and *in vivo* studies are presented whereas the dietary intervention studies are given in chapter 6.

Given the high –albeit sometimes controversial- impact of omega-3 PUFAs on the onset of diseases, this book would look somehow incomplete if the biochemical concept and the scientific evidence of the omega-3 PUFAs supplementation was not given; we do so in chapter 7.

REFERENCES

[1] J. Diamond, *Guns, Germs and Steel, the Fates of Human Societies*, W.W. Norton, New York (1997).

[2] C. D. Mathers and D. Loncar, *PLoS Med.* 3, e442 (2006).

[3] *Global status report on non-communicable diseases 2010.* Geneva, World Health Organization (2011).

[4] *Global atlas on cardiovascular disease prevention and control.* Geneva, World Health Organization (2011).

[5] A. Keys, *A.* Menotti, *C.* Aravanis, H. Blackburn, *B. S.* Djordjevic, R. Buzina, *A. S.* Dontas, F. Fidanza, M. *J.* Karvonen, N. Kimura, I. Mohacek, *S.* Nedeljkovic, V. Puddu, S. Punsar, H. *L.* Taylor, S. Conti, D. Kromhout, *and H.* Toshima, *Prev. Med.* 13, 141 (1984).

[6] A. Menotti, D. Kromhout, H. Blackburn, F. Fidanza, R. Buzina, and A. Nissinen, *Eur. J. Epidemiol.* 15, 507 (1999).

[7] V. L. Roger, A. S. Go, D. M. Lloyd-Jones, E. J. Benjamin, J. D. Berry, W. B. Borden, D. M. Bravata, S. Dai, E. S. Ford, C. S. Fox, H. J. Fullerton, C. Gillespie, S. M. Hailpern, J. A. Heit, V. J. Howard, B. M. Kissela, S. J. Kittner, D. T. Lackland, J. H. Lichtman, L. D. Lisabeth, D. M. Makuc, G. M. Marcus, A. Marelli, D. B. Matchar, C. S. Moy, D. Mozaffarian, M. E. Mussolino, G. Nichol, N. P. Paynter, E. Z. Soliman, P. D. Sorlie, N. Sotoodehnia, T. N. Turan, S. S. Virani, N. D. Wong, D. Woo, and M. B. Turner, *Circulation* 125, 188 (2012).

[8] I. Zabetakis, *J. Food Sci.* 78, R1101 (2013).

[9] *The Mediterranean Diet Pyramid* (last accessed on Oct. 8, 2014). http://dietamediterranea.com/wp-content/uploads/piramide_Eng_logos_DinA4-copy.jpg.

[10] R. Ross, *Nature* 362, 801 (1993).

[11] C. A. Demopoulos, R. N. Pinckard and D. J. Hanahan, *J. Biol. Chem.* 254, 9355 (1979).

[12] C. A. Demopoulos, H. Karantonis and S. Antonopoulou, *Eur. J. Lipid Sci. Tech.* 105, 705 (2003).

[13] C. Nasopoulou, T. Smith, M. Detopoulou, C. Tsikrika, L. Papaharisis, D. Barkas, and I. Zabetakis, *Food Chem.* 145, 1097 (2014).

[14] P. C. Calder and P. Yaqoob, *BioFactors* 35, 266 (2009).

[15] L. Pottel, M. Lycke, T. Bterberg, I. Foubert, H. Pottel, F. Duprez, L. Goethals, and P. R. Debruyne, *Phytochem. Rev.* 1 3, 223 (2014).

[16] J. F. Glatz, T. Borchers, F. Spener, and G. J. van der Vusse, *Prostaglandins Leukot. Essent. Fatty Acids* 52, 121 (1995).

In: Marine Oils (From Sea to Pharmaceuticals) ISBN: 978-1-63463-747-3
Editor: Ioannis Zabetakis

Chapter 5

MARINE OILS AND INFLAMMATION

Constantina Nasopoulou[1,2,*] and Ioannis Zabetakis[2]

[1]Laboratory of Food Chemistry, Faculty of Food Science and Nutrition, School of the Environment, University of the Aegean, Lemnos, Greece

[2]Laboratory of Food Chemistry, Faculty of Chemistry, School of Sciences, National and Kapodistrian University of Athens, Athens, Greece

ABSTRACT

Studies during recent decades have revealed a link between inflammation and nutrition and specific dietary habits seem to alleviate inflammatory processes. Many studies confirm that Mediterranean diet is a dietary pattern that offers protection from the development of some chronic inflammatory diseases such as cardiovascular diseases. Fish is one of the main components of Mediterranean diet, while fish polar lipids (PL) have been found to contain micro constituents with anti-inflammatory properties. The scope of this chapter is to present all resent scientific data regarding fish PL and inflammation.

[*] Corresponding author: Constantina Nasopoulou. Laboratory of Food Chemistry, Faculty of Food Science and Nutrition, School of the Environment, University of the Aegean, Mitr. Ioakim 2, Myrina, 81400, Lemnos, Greece. Laboratory of Food Chemistry, Faculty of Chemistry, School of Sciences, National and Kapodistrian University of Athens, Athens 15771, Greece. E-mail addresses: knasopoulou@aegean.gr; cnasopoulou@chem. uoa.gr.

INTRODUCTION

The human body encounters a huge number of stimuli, on a daily basis many of which result in injuries or infections and damage human cells and tissues leading to lesion development.

In order to overcome such damages, the human body uses inflammation as a response. At a molecular level, this response consists of a series of complex physiological repair pathways catalyzed by specific enzymes [1].

Upon inflammatory response the innate immune cells such as blood leukocytes, mast and dendrite cells are activated. Secreted cytokines such as tumor necrosis factor-a (TNF-a) induce the chemotactic molecules of chemokines to attract the aforementioned immune cells to the site of injury and infection, causing in this way a topic inflammatory condition.

Activated immune cells produce various toxic agents such as reactive oxygen species (ROS), reactive nitrogen species (RNS), elastases, cathepsins, proteinases and platelet activating factor (PAF) (1-O-alkyl-2-acetyl-sn-glycero-3-phosphocholine), that can promote or suppress inflammation. Therefore the rate of inflammation resolution is very critical in order to avoid or limit any damage to host tissue [2].

Mediators of inflammation play an important role in maintaining a balance in an acute inflammatory response. If the initial acute response does not resolve the causative factor then the inflammatory response will continue and the subsequent inflammatory microenvironment will disrupt tissue homeostasis causing a low grade chronic inflammatory condition. This delay or dysregulation of inflammation resolution could be the initiation of a chronic inflammatory disease [3].

Most of the lipid mediators that regulate inflammation are metabolites derived from omega-6 (ω-6) or omega-3 (ω-3) polyunsaturated fatty acids (PUFAS), including arachidonic acid (AA; 20:4ω-6), linoleic acid (LA; 18:2ω-6), eicosapentaenoic acid (EPA; 20:5ω-3), and docosahexaenoic acid (DHA; 22:6ω-3). The ω-6 PUFAs are generally described as pro-inflammatory, while ω-3 PUFAs are generally described as anti-inflammatory. Fish oil (FO) and marine oil (MO), e.g. krill oil, are rich in ω-3 PUFAs, where the proportions of EPA and DHA are predominant. Whether being presented as a part of triacylglycerol molecules, as in FO, or incorporated into phospholipid molecules, as in krill oil, ω-3 PUFAs are capable of influencing different metabolic pathways [4] and modulate physiological effects [5, 6].

The link between dietary PUFA, inflammation and disease susceptibility is partially due to changes in the PUFA content of phospholipids in cells involved in the inflammatory response, such as monocytes, macrophages and vascular endothelial cells [7, 8].

There are scientific data that FO anti-inflammatory properties are mainly attributed to the presence of lipid micro-constituents that act as PAF antagonists either by inhibiting PAF binding to its receptor (PAF-inhibitors) or competing with PAF in binding to its receptor (PAF-agonists) [9-12]. PAF is a potent pro-inflammatory phospholipid mediator that is implicated in the mechanism of atherosclerosis [13]. According to this mechanism, PAF is produced during LDL oxidation [14] and causes in situ inflammation. It is also known that PAF is a compound of atheromatic plaque and is essential for the activation of leukocytes and their binding in the endothelial cells [15].

This chapter aims to analyze the anti-inflammatory properties of FO/MO with emphasize on polar lipids (PL) and omega-3 polyunsaturated fatty acids (PUFAs) focusing on the chronic inflammatory condition of atherosclerosis.

INFLAMMATION

Phospholipids consist of glycerol, usually esterified to a saturated long chain fatty acid at sn-1, to an unsaturated long chain fatty acid at sn-2 and to a phosphorylated head group at sn-3 (Figure 1).

The ω-3 PUFAs, such as the fish origin EPA and DHA PUFAs are incorporated into the sn-2 position of phospholipids in cellular membranes [16].

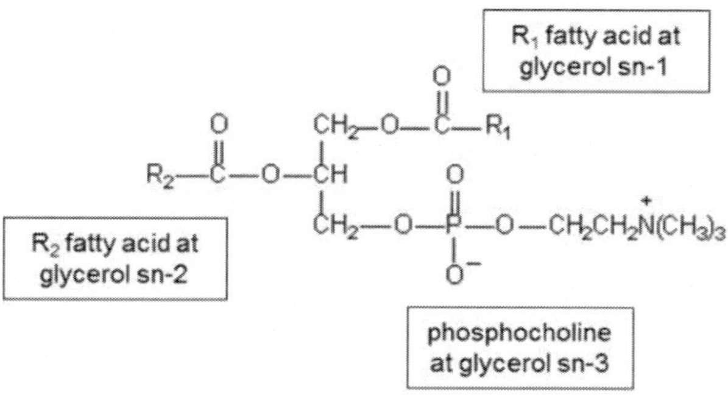

Figure 1. Phospholipids are composed of glycerol, 2 fatty acids esterified to glycerol at sn-1 and sn-2 and a phosphorylated head group esterified at sn-3.

Phospholipid head groups are cytidine-monophosphate, hydroxyl, choline, ethanolamine, serine or inositols [16]. phosphatidylcholine (PC) and phosphatidylethanolamine (PE) are concentrated in macrophage plasma membranes [17] and are the major phospholipids in human plasma (76% PC and 17% PE) [18]. They are also the most abundant phospholipids in human erythrocytes [19]. Therefore, PC and PE are the largest phospholipid reservoirs of dietary ω-6 and ω-3 PUFAs in the cells and biological fluids involved in inflammatory responses.

Other less abundant phospholipids can affect inflammatory responses, but independent of lipid mediator production. For example, diphosphoglycerol (cardiolipin) consisting of 2 molecules of phosphatidic acid esterified to glycerol, is the most abundant phospholipid in the inner mitochondrial membrane [20], can compromise cellular respiration [21] and mediate apoptosis [22] under conditions of oxidative stress.

Another example is PAF, which directly enhances cytokine and adhesion molecules expression in vascular endothelium [23].

EPA and DHA PUFAs are thought to play an important function in the prevention and treatment of cardiovascular, inflammatory and autoimmune diseases, mental disorders, and cancer because of their immunosuppressive action, whereas DHA is crucial for normal functional development of the retina and brain [24].

EPA and DHA are not adequately biosynthesized in humans and other mammals from their precursors linoleic and α-linolenic acids due to the moderate activity of the enzymes involved in their biosynthetic pathway [25-27]. The required amount of these fatty acids appears to be unattainable by this route. Given these biosynthetic complexities and the essential rate of linoleic and α-linolenic acids, it is recommended that they be included in the diet as conditionally essential fatty acids [27].

There is strong evidence that dietary PUFAs influence inflammation response through lipid mediators. For example EPA and DHA dietary supplementation were shown to decrease pro-inflammatory AA-derived eicosanoids, underlining that dietary ω-6 to ω-3 PUFA ratio does in fact influence lipid mediator biosynthesis through changes in PUFA composition of tissue phospholipids [28]. Additionally EPA was associated with a reduction in the systemic macrophage inflammatory response and with increased production of the anti-inflammatory cytokine interleukin-10 (IL-10) [29], while in another study there was a significant decrease in pro-inflammatory markers (IL-6 and TNF-a, $P = 0.0001$) after supplementation of

EPA and DHA [30]. EPA and DHA supplementation could modulate the ability of monocytes to stimulate endothelium [31].

In a double-blinded randomized controlled study in healthy subjects, EPA and DHA dietary supplementation were shown to alter lipid metabolism, increasing the proportion of phospholipids and triglycerides containing long-chain PUFAs [32]. Therefore in vivo production of lipid mediators is regulated by substrate availability.

EPA dietary supplementation to patients awaiting carotid endarterectomy revealed that a higher atherosclerotic plaque EPA content was associated with a reduced number of foam cells and T cells, less inflammation and increased stability [33].

However a meta-analysis of the protective effects of ω-3 PUFA supplementation against human cardiovascular diseases failed to identify any significant health benefits [34] and a randomised, double blind, parallel study in healthy subjects showed that low dose supplementation with EPA and DHA showed no significant difference in pro inflammatory eicosanoids and cytokines; prostaglandin E_2 (PGE_2), thromboxane B_2 (TXB_2), interleukin 1b (IL-1b), tumor necrosis factor alpha (TNFα) [35].

Such inconsistency of the literature could be attributed to the fact that some ω-6 PUFA are substrate for pro-resolving mediators, which can be displaced by ω-3 PUFA supplementation [28]. Additionally, enzymes that synthesize lipid mediators are selective in their use of substrate [36, 37].

On the other hand, supplementation of the entire edible fish tissues of fatty fish (e.g. salmon, rainbow trout, Baltic herring, whitefish, or tuna), has been associated with inflammatory gene expression in peripheral blood mononuclear cells of patients with coronary heart disease, exhibiting decreased AA: EPA ratio in serum lipids, that may induce an anti-inflammatory response at mRNA levels in peripheral blood mononuclear cells [38].

Ischemic Stroke

Post-Ischemic Inflammatory Response

Strokes and heart attacks are the most common clinical results of the chronic inflammatory condition of atherosclerosis. More specifically stroke is caused by the occlusion of a blood vessel by a thrombus or embolism, resulting in an almost immediate loss of oxygen and glucose to the cerebral tissue. Although different mechanisms are involved in the pathogenesis of stroke, increasing evidence shows that ischemic injury and inflammation account for its pathogenic progression [39].

Cerebral ischemia triggers the pathological pathways of the ischemic cascade and ultimately causes irreversible neuronal injury in the ischemic core within minutes of the onset [40].

Several data suggest that inflammatory cells participate in brain tissue remodeling after injury. Microglial cells are the resident macrophages of the brain, playing a crucial role as resident immunocompetent and phagocytic cells in the central nervous system. Oxidative stress caused by the initial ischemic event activates microglia, which can transform into phagocytes and can release a variety of substances many of which are cytotoxic and/or cytoprotective. Additionally there is substantial evidence that activated microglial cells in response to ischemia have the potential of releasing several pro-inflammatory cytokines such as TNF-α, IL-1β, and IL-6, as well as other potential cytotoxic molecules including NO, ROS, and prostanoids [41].

After activation by ischemia, astrocytes, like microglia, are capable of secreting inflammatory factors such as cytokines, chemokines and NO [42]. Cytokines up-regulate the expression of cell adhesion molecules (CAMs). Within four to six hours after ischemia, circulating leukocytes adhere to vessel walls and migrate to the brain with subsequent release of additional pro-inflammatory mediators and causes secondary injury in the penumbra.

Neutrophils are a leukocyte subtype, which secrete cytokines that up-regulate the expression of CAMs and infiltrate the ischemic brain area. Scientific data demonstrated an infiltration of T cells 3 days after the onset of ischemia in a mouse model, along with a production of IL-17 which amplify the inflammatory cascade [43].

Cytokines, Chemokines and Brain Inflammation

Cytokines are a group of small glycoproteins that are produced in response to an antigen and were originally described as mediators for regulating the innate and adaptive immune systems.

Cytokines are thus up-regulated in the brain in a variety of diseases, including stroke. In the brain, cytokines are expressed not only in the cells of the immune system, but are also produced by resident brain cells, including neurons [44]. In addition, it has been shown that peripherally derived cytokines are involved in brain inflammation.

Thus, peripherally derived mononuclear phagocytes, T lymphocytes cells and polymorphonuclear leukocytes produce and secrete cytokines and might contribute to inflammation of the central nervous system [45].

The most studied cytokines related to inflammation in acute ischemic stroke are tumor necrosis factor-α (TNF-α), the interleukins (IL), IL-1β, IL-6, IL-20, IL-10 and transforming growth factor (TGF)-β. IL-1β and TNF-α, appear to exacerbate cerebral injury, while TGF-β and IL-10 could be neuroprotective exerting anti-inflammatory activity [46, 47].

High circulating IL-1β elevates circulating IL-6, another well-known cytokine that is up-regulated following cerebral ischemia [48]. IL-20 is induced when IL-1β modulates the NF-κB pathway, while IL-20 in turn induces the production of IL-6. IL-1 acts via membrane receptors (IL-1R), which can be blocked by a receptor antagonist (IL-1RA).

IL-10 is an anti-inflammatory cytokine that acts by inhibiting IL-1 and TNF-α and by suppressing cytokine receptor expression and receptor activation as well. IL-10 also seems to mediate infarct size reduction by regulatory T cells. Experimental data show that T cells reduce the pro-inflammatory cytokine levels during the early post-ischemic inflammatory phase, while injection of IL-10 in the brain reduces infarct volume [49].

Chemokines, such as, monocyte chemoattractant protein 1 (MCP-1), are a class of cytokines that guide the migration of blood borne inflammatory cells, such as neutrophils and macrophages, towards the source of the chemokine. Consequently, they play important roles in cellular communication and inflammatory cell recruitment. Expression of chemokines, such as MCP-1 and macrophage inflammatory protein-1α (MIP-1α), following focal ischemia is thought to have a deleterious effect by increasing leukocyte infiltration [50].

Platelet Activating Factor (PAF) and Inflammatory Response of Atherosclerosis

PAF, characterized as the glycerylether phospholipid of 1-O-alkyl-2-acetyl-sn-glycero-3-phosphocholine [51], as mentioned before, represents a highly active lipid mediator. It is produced and released by various stimulated cells [52] and promotes through its receptor [53] a wide range of biological responses such as oxidation, inflammation and thrombosis that have been linked to the pathogenesis of many inflammatory chronic diseases [54], such as atherosclerosis [13], cancer [55], renal diseases [56, 57] and diabetes type II [58].

The biosynthesis of PAF is accomplished through two distinctive enzymatic pathways; the de novo pathway; catalyzed by a specific dithiothreitol-insensitive CDP-choline: 1-alkyl-2-acetyl-sn-glycerol choline-phosphotransferase (PAF-cholinephosphotransferase; PAF-CPT, EC 2.7.8.16) that converts 1-O-alkyl-2-acetyl-glycerol to PAF and the remodeling one; catalyzed by lyso-PAF-acetyl-CoA acetyltransferase (Lyso-PAF-acetyl-transferase; Lyso-PAF-AT, EC 2.3.1.67) [59, 60] which acetylates lyso-PAF. A molecular diversity of lyso-PAF-ATs has been identified. One form of PAF-AT is inducible and activated by inflammatory stimulation, while another one is constitutively expressed. Each lyso-PAF-AT biosynthesizes inflammatory and physiological amounts of PAF, depending on the cell type, highlighting in this way the diverse pathological and physiological roles of PAF [61]. Lipid compounds from sea bass (*Dicentrarchus labrax*) and gilthead sea bream (*Sparus aurata*) have been shown to influence the de novo biosynthetic enzyme of PAF (PAF-CPT) in human mesangial cells [62].

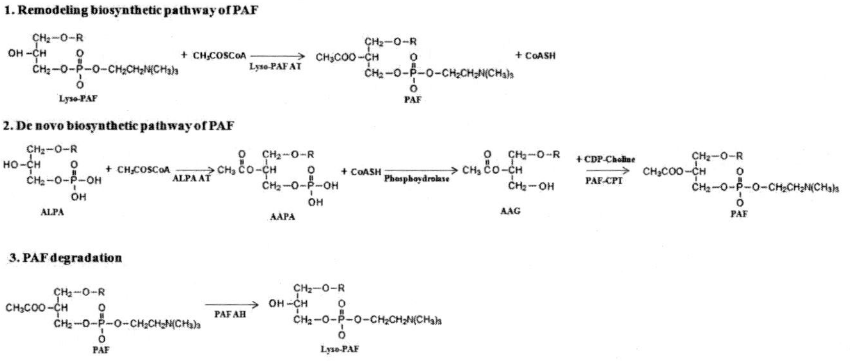

AAG: 1-*O*-alkyl-2-acetyl-glycerol; AAPA: 1-*O*-alkyl-2-acetyl-sn-glycero-3-phosphate; ALPA: 1-*O*-alkyl-sn-glycero-3-phosphate; ALPA AT: 1-*O*-alkyl-sn-glycero-3-phosphate acetyltransferase; AT: acetyltransferase; CDP-choline: cytidine 5-diphosphocholine; Lyso-PAF: Lyso-Platelet Activating Factor; LysoPAF AT: 1-*O*-alkyl-sn-glycero-3-phopshocholine:acetyl-CoA; acetyl-transferase PAF: Platelet Activating Factor; PAF-CPT: PAF-choline-phosphotransferase.

Figure 2. PAF-metabolic pathways.

The catabolism of PAF, to its biologically inactive form, is catalyzed by a PAF specific acetylhydrolase (PAF-AH, EC 3.1.1.47) which plasma form is known as lipoprotein-associated phospholipase A_2 (Lp-PLA_2) [63].

Apart from hydrolysis of the sn-2 acetyl group of PAF, PAF-AH cleaves short chain acyl chains from sn-2 position of oxidized phospholipids known as PAF-like lipids (Figure 2).

More specifically the first pathway or the *remodelling* pathway involves the hydrolysis of pre-existing plasma membrane phospholipids to 1-*O*-alkyl-sn-glycero-3-phosphocholine (lyso-PAF) which is then acetylated by the 1-*O*-alkyl-sn-glycero-3-phopshocholine:acetyl-CoA acetyltransferase (lyso-PAF AT) leading to the formation of PAF. This pathway is responsible for the rapid and increased production of PAF under inflammatory conditions and is mainly regulated by the level and the degree of lyso-PAF AT activation.

The second pathway, defined as the *de novo* pathway, initiates with the acetylation of 1-*O*-alkyl-sn-glycero-3-phosphate (ALPA) by the 1-*O*-alkyl-sn-glycero-3 phosphate acetyl-CoA acetyltransferase (ALPA AT) followed by the sequential action of a phosphohydrolase and a dithiothreitol (DTT)-insensitive cholinephosphotransferase. Unlike the *remodelling* pathway, *de novo* pathway is not activated by inflammatory stimuli but is thought to be responsible for the constitutive production of PAF, maintaining its physiological levels in blood and cells [64, 65].

However, neurotransmitters, such as acetylcholine and dopamine, as well as activators of protein kinase C (PKC) are able to stimulate the synthesis of PAF through the de novo route in chick retina [66] and human endothelial cells [67], respectively, indicating the important regulatory role of the de novo enzymes for the production of PAF.

Several biological activities of PAF indicate the critical role of this lipid mediator in inflammation. PAF stimulates cell mediated active oxygen species production [68], platelet [69] and vascular cells activation [70] and smooth muscle cell growth [71]. It also increases endothelium permeability [68] and promotes angiogenesis [72]. It stimulates the cytokine, chemokine and growth factors release [74] and it is also known as a critical mediator of cell-cell interactions upon inflammation [54, 75].

PAF is produced during LDL oxidation [14], while at the same time its main catabolic enzyme, PAF-AH, exhibits reduced activity in ox-LDL compared with unmodified LDL. In addition, it has been shown that oxygen radicals, that may oxidize LDL, also inhibit Lp-PLA_2 (the plasma form of PAF-AH) [76].

Other studies have shown that Lp-PLA_2 prevents oxidative modification of LDL [77] and further exerts anti-inflammatory activities [78, 79]. Recently, Lp-PLA_2 has been proposed as a biomarker of CVDs [80].

Scientific data indicate that mediators of immunity and inflammation, such as TNF-a and IL-1, stimulate PAF synthesis in human endothelial cells [81]. PAF induces the expression of TNF-a through NF-κB activation [82], while PAF receptor antagonists inhibit IL-1-induced increase in vascular permeability and leukocyte infiltration [83], suggesting a positive feedback network that control the release of PAF, TNF-a and IL-1 [83].

Immune system activation has been recognized as an important condition of chronic inflammatory state implicated in many chronic diseases including atherosclerosis, where toll-like receptors (TLRs), known as key pattern-recognition receptors in innate immunity, play a major role. Scientific evidence show that TLRs are activated not only by exogenous microbial patterns, but also by endogenous factors produced during tissue damage or particle modification that act as TLR ligands and drive inflammation in the absence of infection [84]. Interestingly both PAF and TLR signaling promote noninfectious inflammation through NF-κB activation. Recent studies propose that oxidative modification of molecules such as oxidized phospholipids, known also as PAFlike molecules due to their similarity in structure and activities with PAF, act as TLR ligands, thereby triggering inflammatory responses which form signals that activate TLR-dependent responses [85, 86].

The aforementioned bioactivities indicate that PAF metabolism dysregulation could be a mechanism of inflammatory development at a microenvironment level, which may lead to chronic disease development [13, 87].

Taking into account the critical role of PAF in the inflammatory pathways and based on the beneficial effects of FO/MO on human health it can be hypothesized that FO/MO, beyond their well-studied PUFAs, may have other lipid micro-components that could slow down chronic disease development by down-regulating PAF production and/or enhancing PAF catabolism and/or inhibiting PAF activity at the level of its receptor signaling.

PUFAS WITH ANTI-INFLAMMATORY CAPACITIES

The role of omega-3 polyunsaturated fatty acids (omega-3 PUFAs) against CVDs and other human biological functions has been studied quite extensively in the past (Table 1).

Table 1. Studies on the impact of omega-3 PUFAs [89]

Studied food/compounds	Type of study	Results	References
Consumption of oily fish	Assessing increased levels of omega-3 PUFAs (EPA and DHA)	Favorable cardiovascular prognosis	[90, 91, 92, 93]
Consumption of oily fish at least once a week	Assessing the impact of fish intake to CHD and SCD	50% lower incidence of CHD and SCD	[90, 91, 92, 94]
Supplementation of omega-3 PUFAs (EPA and DHA) to adults	Meta-analysis of 20 studies on 68.680 patients	Omega-3 PUFAs were not statistically significantly associated with CVDs	[34]
Supplementation of omega-3 PUFAs (EPA and DHA)	Review paper summarizing evidence of clinical and animal studies	Omega-3 PUFAs may be linked to cognitive enhancement but further, better designed studies are needed	[95]
Supplementation of omega-3 PUFAs (EPA and DHA)	Assessing the risk of developing ovarian cancer	Neither higher intake of these PUFAs nor the ratio of omega-3 to omega-6 PUFAs was associated with this risk	[96]
Supplementation of omega-3 PUFAs	Influence the production of serum cytokine production and thus depressive symptoms	Omega-3 PUFAs can reduce inflammation in overweight, sedentary middle-aged and older adults	[97]
Omega-3 PUFAs of marine origin	Their role on morbidity of and mortality from CVDs	The impact of omega-3 PUFAs on morbidity of, and mortality from, CVDs is not consistent; further research is needed	[98]

According to United Kingdom's National Health System [88], consumption of oily fish has been linked to higher levels of eicosapentaenoic acid (EPA) and docosahexaenoic acid (DHA) and a subsequent favorable cardiovascular prognosis.

Mechanistically, though, even today, we do not really know how omega-3 PUFAs work. Their postulated mechanism in preventing atherosclerosis could be through lowering the levels of triacylglycerol, preventing arrhythmias, decreasing platelet aggregation, or lowering blood pressure. A possible proarrhythmic effect has been reported but there are still important mechanistic uncertainties that obstruct us in clarifying omega-3 PUFAs' beneficial effects and therefore proving or disproving that there are any clear health benefits of dietary intake of omega-3 PUFAs [99].

Polar Lipids of Marine Oils with Anti-Inflammatory Capacities

Studies during recent decades have revealed a link between inflammation and nutrition and specific dietary habits seem to alleviate inflammatory processes [100]. Many studies confirm that Mediterranean diet is a dietary pattern that offers protection from the development of some chronic inflammatory diseases including CVDs [101] certain types of cancer [102], diabetes [103], metabolic syndrome [104], arthritis [105] and Alzheimer's disease [106].

Recent studies reveal that Mediterranean diet components might have a profound effect on inflammatory response by affecting genetic expression profile. More specifically, the Mediterranean diet including fish and sea food has been associated with decreased expression of genes involved in the inflammatory response [107].

As mentioned before PAF is a potent pro-inflammatory mediator promoting atherosclerosis. In this perspective, the presence of PAF antagonists in fish lipids such as PL (e.g. phospholipids and glycolipids) is very important in terms of cardio-protection.

Rementzis et al. (1997) showed for the first time the presence of PAF antagonists in fish muscle, such as mackerel (*Scomber scombrus*). The lipid components identified in the aforementioned fish muscle were gangliosides and the major one was found to be monosialoganglioside [12]. Gangliosides are complex glycolipids that are found in the outer half of the membrane bilayer and their sugar groups are exposed at the cell surface, suggesting some role in the interactions of the cell with its surroundings. Gangliosides are most abundant in the plasma membrane of nerve cells, where they constitute 5-10% of the total lipids (TL). In most cases, gangliosides occur in free form but there is also evidence indicating their occurrence in complex forms with proteins. These glycolipids as well as their O-acetyl derivatives exhibited important biological activities, such as inducing platelet aggregation through PAF way (PAF-like activity). The presence of lipid constituents with platelet activating properties, such as those found in mackerel does not necessarily mean that they have pro-thrombotic effects since they are five to six orders of magnitude less active than PAF. The presence of such molecules in the bloodstream and their binding to PAF receptors could minimize the biological actions of PAF or in other words they could be considered as PAF inhibitors.

In order to study the effect of frying on biological activity, in terms of platelet activation, of fish lipid fractions (TL, neutral lipids (NL) and PL), the potential aggregatory activity of fresh and fried cod lipids was studied. The obtained results showed that fresh cod lipids (TL, PL and NL) contained both PAF-agonists (PAF-like activity) and PAF-inhibitors whereas fried cod lipids mainly contained PAF-inhibitors [11]. These results suggest that the process of frying can alter fish lipids bioactivity leading to lipids of reduced aggregating activity. These changes are mainly attributed to the absorption of frying medium along with its bioactive substances in the fish [11].

Similar observations, regarding frying, were exhibited in a more recent study conducted on six fish species such as rainbow trout, golden trout, sea bass, herring, coley and plaice [10]. The first three species (rainbow trout, golden trout and sea bass) were farmed while the haddock, coley and plaice had been recently caught from the open sea. The frying medium used was sunflower oil.

All six fish species were examined for the platelet activating properties of their lipid fractions. The obtained results showed that frying led to lipids of reduced aggregatory activity [10]. The biological activity of the lipids extracted from the frying samples could be affected by the absorption of the lipids of the frying medium in the fish flesh, the migration of substances from the fish flesh to the frying medium and from the thermal processing of the sample [108]. A previous study on sunflower oil, revealed that TL, PL and NL of sunflower oil, exhibited inhibitory activities against PAF-induced aggregation [109]. Thus the reduced aggregatory activity of TL, TNL and PL from fried golden trout, rainbow trout and sea bass may be due to the absorption of substances with anti-PAF activities from the sunflower oil.

Additionally, reduction of the amount of the aggregating lipids because of their migration to the frying medium could also be another reason for the decreased aggregatory activity of the frying samples [10].

On the other hand, heating of the samples during frying can lead to alterations in the molecular structure of lipids and thus to alterations of their biological activities. Oxidation and fragmentation are the main chemical changes which take place during heating and several oxidized and fragmented lipid products, such as oxidized phospholipids and cholesterol oxidized products, have been identified in previous studies [110]. Oxidized phospholipids can have potent aggregatory, PAF-like properties [111]. However, in the study conducted by Nomikos at al., 2006 no increase of the aggregatory activity of lipid fractions were found after heating of the samples, probably due to the fact that relatively mild conditions of frying can not induce the formation of such oxidized lipids in fish samples [10].

Regarding the biological activity of farmed and open sea fish species the farmed species exhibited strong aggregatory activities, whereas the open sea species showed mainly inhibitory biological activities [10].

The impact of grilling and brining on the cardio-protective properties of sardine (*Sardina pilchardus*), in terms of PAF-antagonist content, revealed that PL of all specimens (raw, grilled and brined) showed strong inhibitory activity against PAF action, indicating that grilling and brining have not diminished the cardio-protective properties of sardine [112].

A survey performed in order to compare the antiatherogenic properties of lipids obtained from wild and cultured sea bass (*Dicentrarchus labrax*) and gilthead sea bream (*Sparus aurata*) showed that the aggregatory properties of the lipid fractions were dependent on the fish species and whether the fish samples were wild or cultured [9]. Lipid fractions extracted from wild gilthead sea bream showed strong aggregatory properties, while the lipid fractions extracted from farmed fish showed strong inhibitory activities. The aggregatory properties of TL were mainly attributed to PL while the PAF-inhibitory activity was attributed to NL [9]. Similarly lipid fractions extracted from wild sea bass exhibited strong aggregatory properties, while the lipid fractions extracted from farmed fish showed strong PAF-inhibitory activities [9]. The aggregatory properties of sea bass TL were mainly attributed to PL while the PAF- inhibitory activity was attributed to NL [9].

It should be mentioned that all these lipid fractions are a mixture of lipid molecules that can potentially have aggregatory or inhibitory properties. The aforementioned activity observed depends on both the relative ability of each molecule to aggregate platelets or inhibit the PAF-induced platelet aggregation and on the relative amount of each molecule in the mixture. From this perspective a fraction that aggregates platelet may also contain lipid molecules with inhibitory properties and the opposite.

Scientific data has shown that by-products, such as fish brain, are rich in bioactive lipids which are overwhelmingly effective in preventing cardiovascular diseases. Therefore TL were extracted from silver carp (*Hypophthalmichthys molitrix*) brain and separated into PL and NL. The capabilities of the lipid fractions in aggregating washed rabbit platelet or in inhibiting PAF-induced platelet aggregation were tested in order to elucidate the pharmacological activities of silver carp brain lipids against cardiovascular diseases by inhibiting PAF activity [113]. The results showed that the lipid fractions of fish brain exhibited strong inhibitory activities and the activity of TL was mainly attributed to NL [113].

After having reported the presence of PAF antagonists in fish muscle especially in polar lipid class, the in vivo effect of fish PL in atherosclerosis development in diet induced atherosclerosis in male white New Zealand rabbits was studied [114]. More specifically, twelve healthy male New Zealand rabbits of specific weight were randomly divided into two groups of six animals each and were given specific diets for 45 days. Group A was given atherogenic diet 1% cholesterol, while group B was given atherogenic diet enriched with gilthead sea bream PL (0.06% w/w) [114]. The obtained results showed that hypercholesterolemic rabbits that were fed with diet enriched with fish PL, developed early atherosclerosis lesions of significantly lower degree compared with those fed with atherogenic diet (Figure 3) [114].

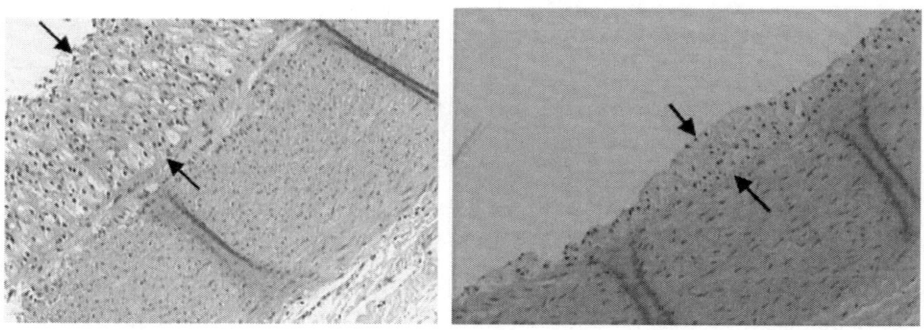

a b

Figure 3. Representative optic micrographs x 100 of aortic wall sections stained with haematoxylin and eosin from the two experimental groups, where atherosclerotic lesions appear as foam cells (↑). (A) Group A (atherogenic diet); (B) Group B (atherogenic diet enriched with gilthead sea bream PL) [114].

This result could be explained on the basis of the elevated PAF-AH activity in the plasma of rabbits of group B in combination with the decreased EC_{50} values of group B. The decreased EC_{50} values of group B could be due to the presence of PAF-inhibitors in gilthead sea bream PL. In addition, earlier scientific data has underlined the in vitro inhibition of PAF-choline-phosphotransferase (PAF-CPT), the main regulatory enzyme of de novo PAF biosynthetic pathway, by gilthead sea bream PL [62].

These results were confirmed by another study that was conducted on the specific activities of four PAF metabolic enzymes, which act in leukocytes, platelets and plasma of the male New Zealand white rabbits of group A and B of the aforementioned *in vivo* experiment [115]. More specifically, the decreased PAF-CPT activity in leukocytes of group B along with the decreased activities of both PAF-CPT and Lyso PAF-AT in platelets of group B have been found to cease further increase on atherosclerotic conditions [115].

References

[1] C. N. Serhan and J. Savill, *Nat. Immunol.* 6, 1191 (2005).
[2] C. Nathan, *Nature* 420, 846 (2002).
[3] R. Medzhitov, *Nature* 454, 428 (2008).
[4] R. J. Deckelbaum, T. S. Worgall and T. Seo, *Am. J. Clin. Nutr.* 83, 1520 (2006).
[5] P. R. Howe, P. M. Clifton and M. J. James, *Lipids* 34, 307 (1999).
[6] T. A. Mori and R. J. Woodman, *Curr. Opin. Clin. Nutr. Metab. Care* 9, 95 (2006).
[7] V. D. F. De Mello, M. Kolehmanien, U. Schwab, L. Pulkkinen, and M. Uusitupa, *Mol. Nutr. Food Res.* 56, 1160 (2012).
[8] W. Raphael and L. M. Sordillo, *Int. J. Mol. Sci.* 14, 21167 (2013).
[9] C. Nasopoulou, T. Nomikos, C. A. Demopoulos, and I. Zabetakis, *Food Chem.* 100, 560 (2007).
[10] T. Nomikos, H. C. Karantonis, C. Skarvelis, C. A. Demopoulos, and I. Zabetakis, *Food Chem.* 96, 29 (2006).
[11] A. Panayiotou, D. Samartzis, T. Nomikos, E. Fragopoulou, H. C. Karantonis, C. A. Demopoulos, and I. Zabetakis, *J. Agric. Food Chem.* 48, 6372 (2000).
[12] J. Rementzis, S. Antonopoulou and C. A. Demopoulos, *J. Agric. Food Chem.* 45, 611 (1997).

[13] C. A. Demopoulos, H. C. Karantonis and S. Antonopoulou, *Eur. J. Lipid Sci. Tech.* 105, 705, (2003).
[14] T. A. Liapikos, S. Antonopoulou, S. A. P. Karabina, D. C. Tsoukatos, C. A. Demopoulos, and A. D. Tselepis, *Biochim. Biophys. Acta* 1212, 353 (1994).
[15] H. W. Mueller, C. A. Haught, J. M. McNatt, K. Cui, S. J. Gaskell, and D. A. Johnston, *Circ. Res.* 77, 54 (1995).
[16] D. E. Vance and J. E. Vance, Phospholipid Biosynthesis in Eukaryotes. In: *Biochemistry of Lipids, Lipoproteins and Membranes,* Vance and Vance, St. Louis, MO, US, (2008).
[17] A. Y. Andreyev, E. Fahy, Z. Guan, S. Kelly, X. Li, J. G. McDonald, S. Milne, D. Myers, H. Park, A. Ryan, et al. *J. Lipid Res.* 51, 2785 (2010).
[18] O. Quehenberger, A. M. Armando, A. H. Brown, S. B. Milne, D. S. Myers, A. H. Merrill, S. Bandyopadhyay, K. N. Jones, S. Kelly, and R. L. Shaner, *J. Lipid Res.* 51, 3299 (2010).
[19] W. Dowhan, M. Bogdanov and E. Mileykovskaya, Functional Roles of Lipids in Membranes. In: *Biochemistry of Lipids, Lipoproteins and Membranes,* Vance and Vance, St. Louis, MO, US, (2008).
[20] G. Paradies, G. Petrosillo, V. Paradies, R. J. Reiter, and F. M. Ruggiero, *J. Pineal Res.* 48, 297 (2010).
[21] A. Musatov and N. C. Robinson, *Free Radic. Res.* 46, 1313 (2012).
[22] H. Yin and M. Zhu, *Free Radic. Res.* 46, 959 (2012).
[23] C. Corl, J. Gandy and L. Sordillo, *J. Dairy Sci.* 91, 3067 (2008).
[24] P. Simopoulos, *J. Am. Coll. Nutr.* 21, 495 (2002).
[25] N. Zamaria, *Reprod. Nutr. Dev.* 44, 273 (2004).
[26] R. Uauy and A. D. Dangour, *Nutr. Rev.* 64, 24 (2006).
[27] L. A. Horrocks and Y. K. Yeo, *Pharmacol. Res.* 40, 211 (1999).
[28] R. C. Poulsen, K. H. Gotlinger, C. N. Serhan, and M. C. Kruger, *Am. J. Hematol.* 83, 437 (2008).
[29] S. Sierra, F. L. Villoslada, M. Comalada, M. Olivares, and J. Xaus. *Nutrition* 24, 245 (2008).
[30] G. B. Perunicic-Pekovic, Z. R. Rasic, S. I. Pljesa, S. S. Sobajic, I. Djuricic, R. Maletic, and D. K. Ristic-Medic, *Nephrology* 12, 331 (2007).
[31] N. T. Luu, J. Madden, P. C. Calder, R. F. Grimble, C. P. Shearman, T. Chan, N. Dastur, W. M. Howell, G. E. Rainger, and G. B. Nash, *J. Nutr.* 137, 2769 (2007).

[32] I. Ottestad, S. Hassani, G. I. Borge, A. Kohler, G. Vogt, T. Hyötyläinen, M. Orešič, K. W. Brønner, K. B. Holven, S. M. Ulven, and M. C. W. Myhrstad, *Plos One* 7, 42550 (2012).
[33] L. Cawood, R. Ding, F. L. Napper, R. H. Young, J. A. Williams, M. J. Ward, O. Gudmundsen, R. Vige, S. P. Payne, S. Ye, et al. *Atherosclerosis* 212, 252 (2010).
[34] E. C. Rizos, E. E. Ntzani, E. Bika, M. S. Kostapanos, and M. S. Elisaf, *JAMA* 308, 1024 (2012).
[35] J. Murphy, K. Galvin, M. Kiely, P. A. Morrissey, N. J. Mann, and A. J. Sinclair, *Asia Pac. J. Clin. Nutr.* 15, 418 (2006).
[36] H. Kühn, J. Belkner, H. Suzuki, and S. Yamamoto, *J. Lipid Res.* 35, 1749 (1994).
[37] H. Kühn, J. Barnett, D. Grunberger, P. Baecker, J. Chow, B. Nguyen, H. Bursztyn-Pettegrew, H. Chan, and E. Sigal, *Biochim. Biophys. Acta.* 1169, 80 (1993).
[38] V. D. F. de Mello, A. T. Erkkilä, U. S. Schwab, L. Pulkkinen, M. Kolehmainen, M. Atalay, H. Mussalo, M. Lankinen, M. Orešič, S. Lehto, et al. *Eur. J. Nutr.* 48, 447 (2009).
[39] W. Muir, P. Tyrrell, N. Sattar, and E. Warburton, *Curr. Opin. Neurol.* 20, 334 (2007).
[40] U. Dirnagl, C. Iadecola and M. A. Moskowitz, *Trends Neurosci.* 22, 391 (1999).
[41] S. M. Lucas, N. J. Rothwell and R. M. Gibson, *Br. J. Pharmacol.* 147, 232 (2006).
[42] R. A. Swanson, W. Ying and T. M. Kauppinen, *Curr. Mol. Med.* 4, 193 (2004).
[43] T. Shichita, Y. Sugiyama, H. Ooboshi, H. Sugimori, R. Nakagawa, I. Takada, T. Iwaki, Y. Okada, M. Iida, D. J. Cua, et al. *Nat. Med.* 15, 946 (2009).
[44] F. C. Barone and G. Z. Feuerstein, *J. Cereb. Blood Flow Metab.* 19, 819 (1999).
[45] C. Ferrarese, P. Mascarucci, C. Zoia, R. Cavarretta, M. Frigo, B. Begni, F. Sarinella, L. Frattola, and M. G. De Simoni, *J. Cereb. Blood Flow Metab.* 19, 1004 (1999).
[46] Y. Zhu, G. Y. Yang, B. Ahlemeyer, L. Pang, X. M. Che, C. Culmsee, S. Klumpp, and J. Krieglstein, *J. Neurosci.* 22, 3898 (2002).
[47] P. A. Spera, J. A. Ellison, G. Z. Feuerstein, and F. C. Barone, *Neurosci. Lett.* 251, 189 (1998).

[48] W. M. Clark, L. G. Rinker, N. S. Lessov, K. Hazel, and F. Eckenstein, *Neurol. Res.* 21, 287 (1999).
[49] A. Liesz, E. Suri-Payer, C. Veltkamp, H. Doerr, C. Sommer, S. Rivest, T. Giese, and R. Veltkamp, *Nat. Med.* 15, 192 (2009).
[50] J. S. Kim, S. C. Gautam, M. Chopp, C. Zaloga, M. L. Jones, P. A. Ward, K. M. A. Welch, *J. Neuroimmunol.* 56, 127 (1995).
[51] C. A. Demopoulos, R. N. Pinckard and D. J. Hanahan, *J. Biol. Chem.* 254, 9355 (1979).
[52] C. Dentan, P. Lesnik, M. J. Chapman, and E. Ninio, *Eur. J. Biochem.* 236, 48 (1996).
[53] S. Ishii and T. Shimizu, *Tanpakushitsu Kakusan Koso* 44, 1068 (1999).
[54] G. A. Zimmerman, T. M. McIntyre, S. M. Prescott, and D. M. Stafforini, *Crit. Care Med.* 30, 294 (2002).
[55] A. B. Tsoupras, C. Iatrou, C. Frangia, and C. A. Demopoulos, *Infect. Disord. Drug Targets* 9, 390 (2009).
[56] N. Lloberas, J. Torras, I. Herrero-Fresneda, J. M. Cruzado, M. Riera, I. Hurtado, J. M. Grinyó, *FASEB J.* 16, 908 (2002).
[57] A. B. Tsoupras, E. Fragopoulou, C. Iatrou, and C. A. Demopoulos, *Curr. Top. Nutraceutical Res.* 9, 105 (2011).
[58] G. B. Kudolo and R. A. DeFronzo, *Prostaglandins Other Lipid Mediat.* 57, 87 (1999).
[59] F. Snyder, *Biochim. Biophys. Acta* 1254, 231 (1995).
[60] F. Snyder, *Biochem. J.* 305, 689 (1995).
[61] T. Harayama, H. Shindou, R. Ogasawara, A. Suwabe, and T. Shimizu, *J. Biol. Chem.* 283, 11097 (2008).
[62] A. B. Tsoupras, E. Fragopoulou, T. Nomikos, C. Iatrou, S. Antonopoulou, and C. A. Demopoulos, *Mediators Inflamm.* 2007, 27683 (2007).
[63] D. M. Stafforini, *Cardiovasc. Drugs Ther.* 23, 73 (2009).
[64] F. Snyder, *Biochem. J.* 305, 689 (1995).
[65] F. Snyder F, *Biochim. Biophys. Acta* 1254, 231 (1995).
[66] F. Bussolino, G. Pescarmona, G. Camussi, and F. Gremo, *J. Neurochem.* 51, 1755 (1988).
[67] R. Heller, F. Bussolino, D. Ghigo, G. Garbarino, G. Pescarmona, and U. Till, *J. Biol. Chem.* 266, 21358 (1991).
[68] P. Bautista and J. J. Spitzer, *Free Radic. Res. Commun.* 17, 195 (1992).
[69] P. Golino, G. Ambrosio, M. Ragni, I. Pascucci, M. Triggiani, A. Oriente, J. McNatt, L. M. Buja, M. Condorelli, M. Chiariello, et al. *Circulation* 88, 1205 (1993).

[70] G. K. Marathe, G. A. Zimmerman, S. M. Prescott, and T. M. McIntyre, *Vascul. Pharmacol.* 38, 193 (2002).
[71] J. M. Heery, M. Kozak, D. M. Stafforini, D. A. Jones, G. A. Zimmerman, T. M. McIntyre, and S. M. Prescott, *J. Clin. Invest.* 96, 2322 (1995).
[72] Y. Jiang, K. Wen, X. Zhou, D. Schwegler-Berry, V. Castranova, and P. He, *Am. J. Physiol. Heart Circ. Physiol.* 295, 898 (2008).
[73] R. Maliba, S. Lapointe, P. E. Neagoe, et al. *Cell Signal* 18, 1947 (2006).
[74] T. W. Kuijpers, B. C. Hakkert, M. H. Hart, and D. Roos, *J. Cell Biol.* 117, 565 (1992).
[75] E. Ninio, S. Leyravaud, J. Bidault, P. Jurgens, and J. Benveniste, *Int. Immunol.* 3, 1157 (1991).
[76] G. Ambrosio, A. Oriente, C. Napoli, G. Palumbo, P. Chiariello, G. Marone, M. Condorelli, M. Chiariello, and M. Triggiani, *J. Clin. Invest.* 93, 2408 (1994).
[77] D. M. Stafforini, G. A. Zimmerman, T. M. McIntyre, and S. M. Prescott, *Trans Assoc. Am. Physicians*, 105, 44 (1992).
[78] L. W. Tjoelker, C. Wilder, C. Eberhardt, D. M. Stafforini, G. Dietsch, B. Schimpf, S. Hooper, H. Le Trong, L. S. Cousens, G. A. Zimmerman, et al. *Nature* 374, 549 (1995).
[79] R. Quarck, G. B. De, D. Stengel, D. Stengel, A. Mertens, M. Lox, G. Theilmeier, C. Michiels, M. Raes, H. Bult, D. Collen, et al. *Circulation* 103, 2495 (2001).
[80] O. Vittos, B. Toana, A. Vittos, and E. Moldoveanu, *Biomarkers* 17, 289 (2012).
[81] F. Bussolino, G. Camussi, C. Tetta, G. Garbarino, A. Bosia, and C. Baglioni, *J. Lipid Mediat.* 2, 15 (1990).
[82] S. Y. Im, S. J. Han, H. M. Ko, J. H. Choi, S. B. Chun, D. G. Lee, T. Y. Ha, and H. K. Lee, *Eur. J. Immunol.* 27, 2800 (1997).
[83] S. Nourshargh, S. W. Larkin, A. Das, T. J. Williams, *Blood* 85, 2553 (1995).
[84] T. Kawai and S. Akira, *Nat. Immunol.* 11, 373 (2010).
[85] E. Mullick, P. S. Tobias and L. K. Curtiss, *J. Clin. Invest.* 115, 3149 (2005).
[86] P. Hodgkinson and S. Ye, *Sci. World J.* 11, 437 (2011).
[87] E. Ninio, *Curr. Opin. Clin. Nutr. Metab. Care* 8, 123 (2005).
[88] *NHS Choices. Fish and shellfish. NHS Live Well.* Available from: http://www.nhs.uk/Livewell/Goodfood/Pages/fish-shellfish.aspx (2011) *(accessed October 14, 2014).*

[89] I. Zabetakis, *J. Food Sci.* 78, R1101 (2013).
[90] K. He, Y. Song, M. L. Daviglus, K. Liu, L. Van Horn, A. R. Dyer, and P. Greenland, *Circulation* 109, 2705 (2004).
[91] S. P. Whelton, J. He, P. K. Whelton, and P. Muntner, *Am. J. Cardiol.* 93, 1119 (2004).
[92] A. Konig, C. Bouzan, J. T. Cohen, W. E. Connor, P. M. Kris-Etherton, G. M. Gray, R. S. Lawrence, D. A. Savitz, and S. M. Teutsch, *Am. J. Prev. Med.* 29, 335 (2005).
[93] *USDA* (US Department of Agriculture, National Nutrition Database for Standard Reference). Release 25. *Available from: http://www.ars.usda.gov/Services/docs.htm?docid=8964 (2012) (accessed October 14, 2014).*
[94] C. M. Albert, C. H. Hennekens, C. J. O'Donnell, U. A. Ajani, V. J. Carey, W. C. Willett, J. N. Ruskin, and J. E. Manson, *JAMA* 279, 23 (1998).
[95] D. W. Luchtman and C. Song, *Neuropharmacology* 64, 550 (2013).
[96] T. I. Ibiebele, C. M. Nagle, C. J. Bain, and P. M. Webb, *Cancer Cause Control* 23, 1775 (2012).
[97] J. K. Kielcolt-Glaser, M. A. Belury, R. Andridge, W. B. Malarkey, B. S. Hwang, and R. Glaser, *Brain Behav. Immun.* 26, 988 (2012).
[98] P. C. Calder and P. Yaqoob, *Curr. Opin. Cardiol.* 27, 412 (2012).
[99] P. Saravanan, N. C. Davidson, E. B. Schmidt, and P. C. Calder, *Lancet* 376, 540 (2010).
[100] D. Giugliano, A. Ceriello and K. Esposito, *J. Am. Coll. Cardiol.* 48, 677 (2006).
[101] F. Sofi, C. Macchi, R. Abbate, G. F. Gensini1, and A. Casini, *BioFactors* 39, 335 (2013).
[102] V. C. La, *Nutr. Rev.* 67, 126 (2009).
[103] K. Esposito, C. M. Kastorini, D. B. Panagiotakos, and D. Giugliano, *Rev. Endocr. Metab. Disord.* 14, 255 (2013).
[104] D. Giugliano and K. Esposito, *Curr. Opin. Lipidol.* 19, 63 (2008).
[105] J. Kjeldsen-Kragh, *Ann. Rheum. Dis.* 62, 193 (2003).
[106] T. Psaltopoulou, T. N. Sergentanis, D. B. Panagiotakos, I. N. Sergentanis, R. Kosti, and N. Scarmeas, *Ann. Neurol.* 74, 580 (2013).
[107] A. Bouchard-Mercier, A. M. Paradis, I. Rudkowska, S. Lemieux, P. Couture, and M. C. Vohl, *Nutr. J.* 12, 24 (2013).
[108] T. Aro, R. Tahvonen, T. Mattila, J. Nurmi, T. Sivonen, and H. Kallio, *J. Agric. Food Chem.* 48, 6085 (2000).
[109] H. C. Karantonis, S. Antonopoulou and C. A. Demopoulos, *J. Agric. Food Chem.* 50, 1150 (2002).

[110] T. Tanaka, A. Tokumura and H. Tsukatani, *Biosci. Biotechnol. Biochem.* 59, 1389 (1995).
[111] A. Tokumura, T. Sumida, M. Toujima, K. Kogure, and K. Fukuzawa, *Biofactors*, 13, 29 (2000).
[112] C. Nasopoulou, E. Psani, E. Sioriki, C. A. Demopoulos, and I. Zabetakis, *Food Nutr. Sci.* 4, 940 (2013).
[113] C. Wang, W. Xia, Y. Xu, Q. Jiang, S. Yin, Y. Yang, and P. Yu, *Lipids Health Dis.* 12, 94 (2013).
[114] C. Nasopoulou, H. C. Karantonis, D. N. Perrea, S. E. Theocharis, D. G. Iliopoulos, C. A. Demopoulos, and I. Zabetakis, *Food Chem.* 120, 831 (2010).
[115] C. Nasopoulou, A. B. Tsoupras, C. H. Karantonis, C. A. Demopoulos, and I. Zabetakis, *Lipids Health Dis.* 10, 213 (2011).

In: Marine Oils (From Sea to Pharmaceuticals) ISBN: 978-1-63463-747-3
Editor: Ioannis Zabetakis

Chapter 6

Dietary Intervention Studies of Fish and FO/MO (Fish Oils/Marine Oils): Focus on Secondary Prevention of Cardiovascular Disease and Diabetes

Paraskevi Detopoulou[1], Elizabeth Fragopoulou[2], Tzortzis Nomikos[2] and Smaragdi Antonopoulou[2,*]

[1]Department of Nutrition, General Hospital
Korgialenio Benakio, Athens, Greece
[2]Department of Nutrition-Dietetics,
Harokopio University, Athens, Greece

Abstract

A systematic study of the literature on the secondary prevention of cardiovascular disease and diabetes was performed including studies with hard clinical end-points. With regard to cardiovascular disease, ten studies were identified, from which the majority focus on fish oil administration rather than fish intake and are based mostly on men. Early studies on omega-3 fatty acids (DART-1, GISSI, GISSI-HF, JELIS) have shown beneficial results with some exceptions (DART-2, Nielsen et al. 2001). However, in most (Alpha-Omega Trial, Omega, SU.FOL.OM3) but not all recent studies (Poole et al., 2013) fish oils were ineffective in

[*] Corresponding author: Smaragdi Antonopoulou. E-mail address: antonop@hua.gr.

secondary prevention. A possible explanation for this difference is the increase of statins prescription, which may mask the effects of fish oils. As far as studies in patients with diabetes are concerned, only two studies were identified (Poole et al., 2013 and ORIGIN) with the first showing a protective effect of fish oils in all- cause mortality and the second showing no effect on death or other cardiovascular outcome. To sum up, the available data are not yet sufficient to support any supplementation of fish oils for the prevention of cardiovascular disease in patients who have already had a cardiovascular event or diabetes. In this context, the joint statement of the European Society of Cardiology (ESC) and the European Association for the Study of Diabetes (EASD) clearly underlines the importance of omega-3 fatty acids (2–4 g/day) for triacylglycerol lowering but not for risk reduction.

INTRODUCTION

Despite the on-going advances in technology and science, cardiovascular disease and diabetes remain a constantly growing epidemic, which not only increases the risk for mortality, but also imposes a serious economic burden [1]. Indeed, the overall healthcare expenditure for cardiovascular disease [2] and diabetes [1] is estimated at 196 billion and 75 billion Euros per year, respectively and is expected to increase [1]. The alarming statistics highlight the need for effective strategies to combat these chronic diseases.

Diet and physical activity constitute cornerstones for the prevention and management of cardiovascular disease and diabetes [1]. In this context, several foods and dietary supplements have been tested, among which are fish, fish oils and marine oils. The interest in fish and related oils has arisen from early observations of Greenland Eskimos, who traditionally consume large amounts of fish [3] and have a low prevalence of cardiovascular disease and diabetes [4, 5]. This observation was corroborated by the results of the Seven Countries Study, which demonstrated that Japanese, who have a high fish intake, suffer less from cardiovascular disease [6]. Recently, the omega-3 index (red blood cell membrane EPA and DHA) has emerged as a potential risk marker for cardiovascular disease [7].

A plethora of studies have documented the cardioprotective effects of fish and fish oils in various experimental conditions (animal studies, observational studies and clinical trials) [8]. Moreover, evidence from animal and *in vitro* studies support an insulin-sensitizing action of EPA and DHA [9, 10]. Since etiological relations can be established through clinical studies, it is the intent of this chapter to present a systematic literature review on the intervention studies with fish/marine oils with a special focus on secondary prevention of cardiovascular disease and diabetes, which is considered an equivalent of cardiovascular disease [11]. Studies with hard clinical end-points were included, i.e. all-cause mortality, cardiovascular mortality, myocardial infarction or other cardiovascular episodes.

DIETARY INTERVENTION STUDIES ON PATIENTS WITH CARDIOVASCULAR DISEASE

Several clinical trials have been carried out for the secondary prevention of cardiovascular disease with fish or fish oils (Table 1). The conducted studies on patients with cardiovascular disease enrolled ~ 51.600 patients aged 60-70 years in total, who received 0.4- 4 g of fish oils for 1- 9 years. Briefly, the first study investigating the effect of fish or fish oils on secondary prevention of cardiovascular disease was the DART study (Diet And Reinfarction Trial) [12]. In this study, patients were instructed to eat 2 portions of fish per week (200-400 g) or 0.5 g omega-3 fatty acids if fish consumption was not possible. After a 2-year follow-up total mortality had been reduced by 29% [12]. Some years later, the same study group conducted a similar study on 3,000 patients with angina (DART-2), in which the opposite results were found (26% increase of mortality after 9 year follow-up) [13]. The investigators attributed the results to the low adherence of the participants to the diet. The GISSI Study (Gruppo Italiano per lo Studio della Sopravvivenza nell Infarto miocardico) included 11,000 patients, who took a supplement of omega-3 fatty acids within 4 months after the onset of myocardial infraction containing (850–882 mg EPA + DHA), vitamin E (300 mg), both, or nothing (control group) [14]. After a 3.5 year follow-up, the omega-3 group experienced less cardiovascular events while the vitamin E group had no beneficial effect. In the GISSI-Heart Failure study (GISSI- HF) 7,046 patients with heart failure participated and took 1 g of omega-3 fatty acids per day [15]. The results were beneficial for total mortality.

In the JELIS study (Japan Eicosapentaenoic acid (EPA) Lipid Intervention Study) 18.645 Japanese subjects with hypercholesterolemia (70% women) were randomized in two groups: one group taking 1.800 mg EPA per day with statin (EPA group, n~9,000) or only statin (control group, n~9,000) [16]. Subjects with myocardial infarction in the last 6 months were excluded.

Patients were followed-up after 5 years and a reduction in cardiovascular events was evident (19% reduction in major cardiovascular events). In a sub-analysis of patients with known heart disease (n~3,450 subjects) a reduction of coronary events was observed (↓ 8.7%). It is noted that participants of the JELIS study had a high background intake of omega-3 fatty acids through fish intake.

In the study of Nielsen et al. a high dose of omega-3 was administered (4 g per day) but no beneficial effect was observed, possibly because of the small sample size [17]. In the Alpha Omega Trial 4,837 cardiovascular patients were included (78% men), who had had a history of myocardial infraction in the last 4 years [18]. The patients were administered 400 mg EPA + DHA or 2 g ALA (in the form of margarine), a combination of two, or placebo and patients were followed up for 3.3 years. The administration of EPA+DHA alone or in combination with ALA did not lead to cardiovascular events reduction, with an exception of the subgroup of women in which a trend for CVD reduction was noticed after the omega-3 administration (P=0.07). The absence of beneficial effects of omega-3 in this study may be due to the low doses administered and/or the parallel statin treatment.

It is noted that the margarine administered had 2.3 times more ω-6 fatty acids than those in the Lyon study. According to a sub-analysis of the Alpha Omega trial patients, those with cardiovascular disease who were not treated with statins (n =413 non stastin users vs n=3,740 statin users) had fewer cardiovascular events than statin users [19].

In the Omega trial, 1 g/d of omega-3 fatty acids were given (460 mg EPA +380 mg DHA) to 3,851 patients (74 % men) shortly after the onset of myocardial infarction (3-14 days after the case) [20]. The patients were followed up after 1 year and no difference was observed between groups. This result may be due to statin intake and/or the increase in fish intake throughout the study. Moreover, the study may be underpowered, since the number of death events was lower than expected due to improved treatment.

In the SU.FOL.OM3 study, 1863 patients with cardiovascular disease were treated with 600 mg/day omega-3 or vitamin B for a period of 4.2 years; none of the interventions in the SU.FOL.OM3 study had beneficial effects on cardiovascular outcomes [21].

To sum up, the majority of studies conducted so far have focused mostly on fish oil and not fish intake. In particular, only two studies have examined the effects of fish intake on cardiovascular outcomes on high-risk patients having controversial results [12, 13]. Another point that should be mentioned is that in studies with omega-3/statin intake men were mostly represented, while in the JELIS study, in which women were over-represented beneficial effects were observed [16]. It is worth noting that earlier studies on omega-3 fatty acids showed positive results while recent studies, in which most participants took statins, have not shown beneficial effects [18, 20].

Several recent meta-analysis also stress the same issue. One from Kwake et al. including 20.485 patients with cardiovascular disease concluded that omega-3 fatty acids did not reduce the risk of cardiovascular events (RR: 0.99; 95% CI: 0.89–1.09) [22]. Another meta-analysis from Rizos et al. including 68,680 patients similarly showed no beneficial results for cardiac death, myocardial infarction and stroke [23].

With regard to the masking effect of statins, several mechanisms have been proposed. First, statins may alter the omega-6/omega-3 ratio, since they increase arachidonic acid [24, 25]. Given the competition of the omega-6/omega-3 series from a biochemical point of view, in a different polyunsaturated fatty acid milieu with plenty of omega-6, omega-3 fatty acids may not exhibit their protective effects [26]. Another possible direction of statins/omega-3 interplay involves mitochondria. On one hand, omega-3 fatty acids improve mitochondrial function and may stimulate myocardial preconditioning [27, 28], which is a physiological mechanism that reduces the extent of cell death after an ischemic episode. On the other hand, statins exhibit a dose- depending toxic effect at mitochondria level [29, 30]. Given the critical role of mitochondria in myocardial preconditioning [31] and its importance for patients with cardiovascular disease, this means that statins could impair the beneficial effects of omega-3 fatty acids in this high-risk group. Last but not least, results from our group have shown that statins behave as PAF inhibitors while simvastatin also suppresses *de novo* PAF-biosynthesis in leukocytes of healthy volunteers [32]. In parallel, omega-3 fatty acids and fish exhibit a PAF-inhibitory activity [33-35], which constitute one of their potential beneficial mechanistic aspects. The co-ingestion of statins and fish oils, which share selected molecular targets, may reduce the efficacy of the latter. It is noted that smaller studies assessing the extent of restenosis or the diameter of atherosclerotic coronary arteries after omega-3 supplementation have not shown any beneficial effect [36, 37].

More studies are required to understand the role of fish oils when administered together with guideline-adjusted treatment, such as statins, in large patient populations. The ongoing REDUCE-IT Study (Reduction in Cardiovascular Events with EPA-Intervention Trial, REDUCE-IT; NCT01492361) will evaluate the effect of purified EPA (4 g/day) on cardiovascular outcomes in high-risk patients under statin therapy [38].

The need for the study of the interaction of diet with statin therapy has also been highlighted in recent guidelines for cardiovascular disease by the American Heart association [11].

Dietary Intervention Studies on Patients with Diabetes

The studies investigating the effects of fish oils on cardiovascular outcomes of patients with type 2 diabetes are summarized in Table 2. The conducted studies in diabetes are numerous (29 studies) but quite heterogeneous since the administered doses of fish oil ranged from 1 to 10 g and the duration of the studies was from 2 months to 6.7 years, with the highest supplementation period in the recently completed ORIGIN Study. Most of them are relatively small studies with a sample of 10-50 patients taking fish oils for a period of 8-12 weeks.

It is noteworthy that most studies on patients with diabetes lack hard cardiovascular endpoints, with the exception of the ORIGIN Study. In that study 12,536 patients with diabetes participated from 573 centers in 40 countries [39]. They were given 1g fish-oil capsules, which contained 465 mg EPA and 375 mg DHA. After a 6-year follow-up no beneficial effect was shown on death or other cardiovascular outcome [39].

An ongoing study may shed more light on the role of fish oils in diabetes patients. The ASCEND Study (A Study of Cardiovascular Events in Diabetes, NCT00135226) will enroll 15,480 participants with diabetes, randomize them to 1 g of omega-3 fatty acids or placebo and assess the incidence of cardiovascular events. The follow-up of the study's participants will be completed by 2017.

Potential Mechanisms of Action

Omega-3 fatty acids have beneficial effects on heart rate, blood pressure, platelet aggregation, inflammatory burden and the reduction of triacylglycerol levels [8]. Doses of omega- 3 fatty acids in the range of 3-4 g/ day lower triacylglycerols by 30-40 % [40] while they do not affect the levels of total and LDL-C [8].

Table 1. Studies investigating the effect of omega-3 or fish intake on secondary prevention of cardiovascular diasease

No	Study	n, duration	Mean age (y)	Country	Start of therapy	Fish	Fish oils	Outcome
1	DART [12]	n=2,033 2 y	61	Great Britain	4 months	2 times/week	-	↓ mortality (30%) ↓ cardiovascular mortality (16 %)
2	DART 2 [13]	n=3,000 9 y	61	Great Britain	†	2 times/week	-	↑ mortality (26%)
3	GISSI [14]	n=11,323 3.5 y	59	Italy	< 3 months	-	1 g ω-3 (0.85–0.88 g EPA + DHA)	↓ mortality (20%) ↓ cardiovascular mortality (30%)
4	GISSI-HF [15]	n=7,046 3.9 y	67	Italy	na	-	1 g EPA+DHA	~ ↓ mortality and cardiovascular mortality (10%)
5	JELIS [16, 82]	n=18,645 hyper-cholesterolemic patiets (n=3,664 patients with CVD) 4.6 y	61	Japan	na	-	1.8 g EPA	↓ mortality (20%) ↓ major coronary events in patients with prior CVD
6	Nielsen et al. [17]	n=300 1-2 y	64	Norway	immediately	-	4 g	ns
7	Alpha-Omega Trial [18, 19]	n=4.837 10 y	69	Holland	4 years	-	0.4 g EPA + DHA 2 g ALA	ns in patients without statin treatment ↓ cardiovascular events

Table 1. (Continued)

No	Study	n, duration	Mean age (y)	Country	Start of therapy	Fish	Fish oils	Outcome
8	Omega [20]	n=3.851 1 y	64	Germany	3-14 days	-	1 g	ns
9	SU.FOL.OM3 [83]	n=572 4.7 y	60	France	< 12 months	-	0.6 g EPA + DHA (ratio 2:1)	ns
10	Poole et al. [84]	n=2,466 patients (1,609 patients with diabetes)	63 (for patients without diabetes)	United Kingdom	90 or 14 days after MI	-	1 g	↓ all- cause mortality in all groups

ns: non significant. na: not available. †In this study patients had angina and the time interval from CVD episode cannot be calculated.

Table 2. Studies investigating the effect of omega-3 on patients with type 2 diabetes

No	Study	N Duration	Mean age or age range (y)	Country	Start of therapy	Fish oils	Outcome	Comments
1	Poole et al. [84]	2,466 patients (1,609 patients with diabetes)	67 (for patients with diabetes)	United Kingdom	90 or 14 days after MI	1 g	↓ all- cause mortality in all groups	patients with diabetes and previous MI
2	ORIGIN [39]	12,536 6.2 years	64	573 centers in 40 countries		1 g highly purified capsules (465 mg EPA + 375 mg DHA)	No effect on death or other cardiovascular outcome	Subjects with impaired fasting glucose, impaired glucose tolerance, or diabetes were included. ~60% of patients had an MI, stroke, or revascularization

MI: Myocardial Infarction.

Studies investigating an alternative source of DHA from microalgae have documented a moderate increase in HDL and LDL-C [41, 42]. The hypotriglyceridemic mechanism of action of omega-3 fatty acids involves the activation of the nuclear peroxisome proliferator-activated receptors (PPARs) [43]. The binding of omega-3 fatty acids with the above receptors regulate the expression of genes encoding proteins involved in fatty acid metabolism (e.g. increase of beta- oxidation in the liver) and synthesis of VLDL and triacylglycerols in the liver (decrease triacylglycerols biosynthesis) [43]. It is noted that co-administration of omega-3 and statins leads to further improvement in the lipid profile compared to statin alone, which indicates that statins and omega-3 influence lipid metabolism through distinct routes [44].

Early studies using large amounts of fish oil (~ 5-10 g/day) reported unfavorable effects on the glycemic profile of patients with type 2 diabetes [45-47]. However, lower intake of fish oils (1-2 g omega-3) do not seem to negatively influence glycemia in subjects with type 2 diabetes [48], while in one study insulin sensitivity was improved [49].

Omega-3 fatty acids may reduce blood pressure in patients with hypertension and hypercholesterolemia [50], probably due to changes in the physicochemical properties of cell membranes, reduced vascular tone [51, 52] and release of nitric oxide [53]. Moreover, fish -oils reduce heart rate [54-57], and improve ventricular function in humans [54, 58, 59] possibly by increasing the elastic properties of myocardial cells [59] and the production of nitric oxide [60]. Interestingly, some clinical trials suggest a differential action of EPA and DHA, with DHA possibly having more protective effects [61]. In parallel, their cardioprotective action involves a more efficient mitochondrial function and production of ATP [62]. Their anti-arrhythmic action has been shown in animals but in humans the available data is not clear [8].

The antithrombotic effect of omega -3 fatty acids are probably mediated by the reduction of thromboxanes (TXA2) [63], a reduction of the expression of platelet derived growth factors -A and -B [64] and PAF production [65] and/or inhibition [33, 34]. According to a recent meta-analysis including 15 studies omega-3 reduced ADP- induced platelet aggregation (standard mean difference -1.23 with 95% confidence interval from -2.24 to -0.23, P=0.02), with the effects being more prominent in patients with cardiovascular disease and diabetes [66]. As far as the *in vitro* anti-inflammatory action of omega-3 fatty acids is concerned, it depends on their involvement in many molecular pathways and their effects on the physico-chemical composition of cell membranes, the function of transcription factors such as NF-κB and the expression of eicosanoids of series 3 and 5 [8].

In his recent review Philip Calder underlines that omega-3 reduce leukocyte chemotaxis and the expression of adhesion molecules and inflammatory cytokines, decrease T-cell reactivity and increase the production of resolvins and protectins [67]. In addition, some components of fish oils (other than omega-3) have anti-atherogenic properties through their ability to inhibit the biological actions of PAF [33, 34].

The results of randomized clinical trials are not as promising as those of the *in-vitro* studies. Indeed, according to a systematic review of 10 randomized clinical trials, omega-3 fatty acids do not have a significant effect on CRP and other indices of inflammation, such as cytokines and chemokines in healthy subjects with some exceptions [68].

Randomized clinical trials in patients with cardiovascular disease (n=7 studies) have shown similar results [68] but in some studies circulating CRP [69], IL-6 [69, 70] and TNF-a were reduced [70].

Considerations: Fish or Fish Oil?

Although few intervention studies have tested the effects of fish on patients with cardiovascular disease and diabetes, before choosing between fish and fish oils several issues should be considered (Figure 1). Fish contain many other nutrients except omega-3 fatty acids, such as vitamin A, D, B_{12}, iron, iodine, selenium, zinc and essential amino acids [71]. Moreover, the bioavailability of several nutrients may be higher in fish compared to fish oils. For example, selenium status is improved to a greater extent by the consumption of salmon rather than salmon oil [72]. Similarly EPA/DHA from fish may be better absorbed from fish than fish oils as a result of interaction with other fats found in fish [73, 74]. Safety issues regarding fish intake include its mercury and polychlorinated biphenyls content [71]. For this reason it is recommended that vulnerable populations, and mainly pregnant women and young children, should consume less than 2 meals of fatty fish per week (such as tuna and salmon) and avoid shark, swordfish, king mackerel and tilefish [75]. As far as the risk of exposure to polychlorinated biphenyls is concerned, it is similar to other foods, such as meat and dairy products [76]. In total, after weighing up the potential harms and benefits of fish consumption, it is concluded that 2 servings per week outweigh the potential hazards [71].

Furthermore, fish oils have also problematic aspects. Chemical analysis of fish oil supplements have demonstrated that the existent omega-3 fatty acid content was not fully comparable to that stated on the label, with differences ranging from less than 20% to more than 80% of the labeled concentrations [77, 78]. According to a recent publication of EFSA, EPA plus DHA at doses up to 5 g/day or EPA alone up to 1.8 g/day, are considered safe [79]. Although the risk of bleeding is low in such quantities [80], a recent case report from our group seems alarming [81]. We reported a case of an amateur athlete, who consumed about 20 g omega-3 fatty acids per day for a period of one year together with other natural supplements (such as spirulina, hippophae, aloe vera etc). This man presented in hospital with duodenum ulcer and bleeding after the co-ingestion of cortisone and antibiotics [81]. Such cases bring awareness about the potential adverse reactions of supplements in high doses when combined with medications.

Conclusion

Multiple biochemical aspects related to cardiovascular disease and diabetes may be affected by omega-3 fatty acids, such as lipid profile, blood pressure, inflammation and platelet aggregation. However, the evidence from clinical trials lends little support for any favorable effects of omega-3 fatty acids in secondary prevention of cardiovascular disease and diabetes control. The role of omega-3 treatment should be viewed under the prism of Hippocrates words "primum nil nocere", which means "first, do no harm".

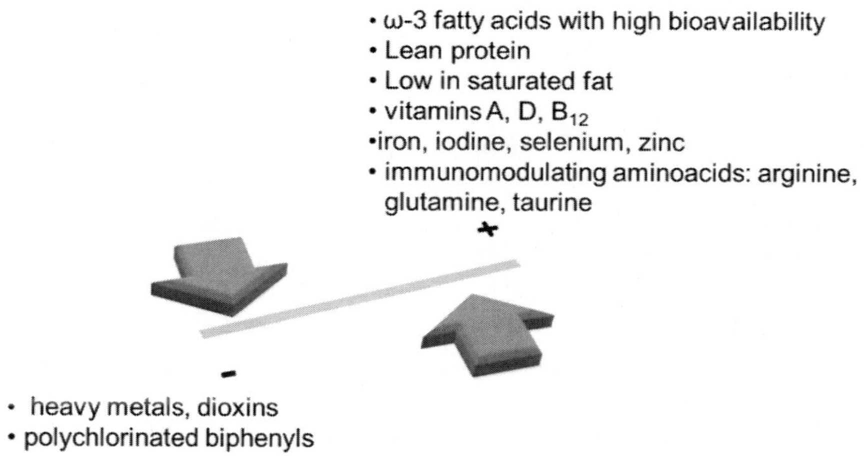

Figure 1. Risks and benefits of fish intake.

In other words, there is no conclusive proof of their efficacy yet, at least as far as secondary prevention of cardiovascular disease and diabetes are concerned.

Taking into account recent evidence, the joint statement of the European Society of Cardiology (ESC) and the European Association for the Study of Diabetes (EASD) clearly underlines the importance of omega-3 fatty acids (2–4 g/day) for triacylglycerol lowering but not for risk reduction [1]. In line with this, the American Heart Association has recently recommended that a healthy eating pattern rich in foods with lean protein, such as fish, fruit, vegetables and low in sodium may be a more effective strategy to combat chronic diseases than single nutrients [11]. Until more data from clinical trials are available no clear recommendation can be made for routine fish oil therapy so… "let fish be your medicine".

REFERENCES

[1] L. Ryden, P. J. Grant, S. D. Anker, C. Berne, F. Cosentino, N. Danchin, C. Deaton, J. Escaned, H. P. Hammes, H. Huikuri, M. Marre, N. Marx, L. Mellbin, J. Ostergren, C. Patrono, P. Seferovic, M. S. Uva, M. R. Taskinen, M. Tendera, J. Tuomilehto, P. Valensi, J. L. Zamorano, S. Achenbach, H. Baumgartner, J. J. Bax, H. Bueno, V. Dean, C. Erol, R. Fagard, R. Ferrari, D. Hasdai, A. W. Hoes, P. Kirchhof, J. Knuuti, P. Kolh, P. Lancellotti, A. Linhart, P. Nihoyannopoulos, M. F. Piepoli, P. Ponikowski, P. A. Sirnes, J. L. Tamargo, A. Torbicki, W. Wijns, S. Windecker, G. De Backer, E. A. Ezquerra, A. Avogaro, L. Badimon, E. Baranova, J. Betteridge, A. Ceriello, C. Funck-Brentano, D. C. Gulba, J. K. Kjekshus, E. Lev, C. Mueller, L. Neyses, P. M. Nilsson, J. Perk, Z. Reiner, N. Sattar, V. Schachinger, A. Scheen, H. Schirmer, A. Stromberg, S. Sudzhaeva, M. Viigimaa, C. Vlachopoulos, R. G. Xuereb, *Eur. Heart. J.* 34, 3035 (2013).

[2] M. Nichols, N. Townsend, R. Luengo-Fernandez, J. Leal, A. Gray, P. Scarborough, M. Rayner, "European Cardiovascular Disease Statistics 2012" *Report of the European Society of Cardiology*, Brussels, Sophia Antipolis (2012).

[3] H. O. Bang, J. Dyerberg, H. M. Sinclair, *Am. J. Clin. Nutr.* 33, 2657 (1980).

[4] N. Kromann and A. Green, *Acta Med. Scand.* 208, 401 (1980).

[5] G. J. Mouratoff, N. V. Carroll, E. M. Scott, *JAMA*, 199, 107 (1967).

[6] A. Menotti, D. Kromhout, H. Blackburn, F. Fidanza, R. Buzina, A. Nissinen, *Eur. J. Epidemiol.* 15, 507 (1999).

[7] C. von Schacky, *Prost. Other Lipid Mediat.* 96, 94 (2011).

[8] D. Mozaffarian and J. H. Wu, *J. Am. Coll. Cardiol.* 58, 2047 (2011).

[9] Y. B. Lombardo, G. Hein, A. Chicco, *Lipids* 42, 427 (2007).

[10] G. Andersen, K. Harnack, H. F. Erbersdobler, V. Somoza, *Ann. Nutr. Metab.* 52, 250 (2008).

[11] R. H. Eckel, J. M. Jakicic, J. D. Ard, V. S. Hubbard, J. M. de Jesus, I. M. Lee, A. H. Lichtenstein, C. M. Loria, B. E. Millen, N. H. Miller, C. A. Nonas, F. M. Sacks, S. C. Smith, Jr., L. P. Svetkey, T. W. Wadden, S. Z. Yanovski, *Circulation,* in press (2013).

[12] M. L. Burr, A. M. Fehily, J. F. Gilbert, S. Rogers, R. M. Holliday, P. M. Sweetnam, P. C. Elwood, N. M. Deadman, *Lancet*, 2, 757 (1989).

[13] M. L. Burr, P. A. Ashfield-Watt, F. D. Dunstan, A. M. Fehily, P. Breay, T. Ashton, P. C. Zotos, N. A. Haboubi, P. C. Elwood, *Eur. J. Clin. Nutr.* 57, 193 (2003).

[14] R. Marchioli, F. Barzi, E. Bomba, C. Chieffo, D. Di Gregorio, R. Di Mascio, M. G. Franzosi, E. Geraci, G. Levantesi, A. P. Maggioni, L. Mantini, R. M. Marfisi, G. Mastrogiuseppe, N. Mininni, G. L. Nicolosi, M. Santini, C. Schweiger, L. Tavazzi, G. Tognoni, C. Tucci, F. Valagussa, *Circulation*, 105, 1897 (2002).

[15] L. Tavazzi, A. P. Maggioni, R. Marchioli, S. Barlera, M. G. Franzosi, R. Latini, D. Lucci, G. L. Nicolosi, M. Porcu, G. Tognoni, *Lancet*, 372, 1223 (2008).

[16] M. Yokoyama, H. Origasa, M. Matsuzaki, Y. Matsuzawa, Y. Saito, Y. Ishikawa, S. Oikawa, J. Sasaki, H. Hishida, H. Itakura, T. Kita, A. Kitabatake, N. Nakaya, T. Sakata, K. Shimada, K. Shirato, *Lancet* 369, 1090 (2007).

[17] D. W. Nilsen, G. Albrektsen, K. Landmark, S. Moen, T. Aarsland, L. Woie, *Am. J. Clin. Nutr.* 74, 50 (2001).

[18] D. Kromhout, E. J. Giltay, J. M. Geleijnse, *N. Engl. J. Med.* 363, 2015 (2010).

[19] S. R. Eussen, J. M. Geleijnse, E. J. Giltay, C. J. Rompelberg, O. H. Klungel, D. Kromhout, *Eur. Heart. J.* 33, 1582 (2012).

[20] B. Rauch, R. Schiele, S. Schneider, F. Diller, N. Victor, H. Gohlke, M. Gottwik, G. Steinbeck, U. Del Castillo, R. Sack, H. Worth, H. Katus, W. Spitzer, G. Sabin, J. Senges, *Circulation* 122, 2152 (2010).

[21] P. Galan, E. Kesse-Guyot, S. Czernichow, S. Briancon, J. Blacher, S. Hercberg, *BMJ* 341, c6273 (2010).

[22] S. M. Kwak, S. K. Myung, Y. J. Lee, H. G. Seo, *Arch. Intern. Med.* 172, 686 (2012).

[23] E. C. Rizos, E. E. Ntzani, E. Bika, M. S. Kostapanos, M. S. Elisaf, *JAMA* 308, 1024 (2012).

[24] M. de Lorgeril, P. Salen, A. Guiraud, S. Zeghichi, F. Boucher, J. de Leiris, *Nutr. Metab. Cardiovasc. Dis.* 15, 36 (2005).

[25] P. Rise, S. Ghezzi, I. Priori, C. Galli, *Biochem. Pharmacol.* 69, 1095 (2005).

[26] C. E. Ramsden, J. R. Hibbeln, S. F. Majchrzak, J. M. *Br. J. Nutr.* 104, 1586 (2010).

[27] R. J. Khairallah, K. M. O'Shea, B. H. Brown, N. Khanna, C. Des Rosiers, W. C. Stanley, *J. Pharmacol. Exp. Ther.* 335, 155 (2010).

[28] J. B. McMillin, R. J. Bick, C. R. Benedict, *Am. J. Physiol.* 263, H1479 (1992).

[29] Y. L. Dai, T. H. Luk, C. W. Siu, K. H. Yiu, H. T. Chan, S. W. Lee, S. W. Li, S. Tam, B. Fong, C. P. Lau, H. F. Tse, *Cardiovasc. Toxicol.* 10, 130 (2010).

[30] P. Kaufmann, M. Torok, A. Zahno, K. M. Waldhauser, K. Brecht, S. Krahenbuhl, *Cell Mol. Life Sci.* 63, 2415 (2006).

[31] D. R. Schwartz and M. N. Sack, *Curr. Opin. Pharmacol.* 8, 160 (2008).

[32] N. Tsantila, A. B. Tsoupras, E. Fragopoulou, S. Antonopoulou, C. Iatrou, C. A. Demopoulos, *Angiology*, 62, 209 (2011).

[33] A. Panayiotou, D. Samartzis, T. Nomikos, E. Fragopoulou, H. C. Karantonis, C. A. Demopoulos, I. Zabetakis, *J. Agric. Food Chem.* 48, 6372 (2000).

[34] C. Nasopoulou, T. Nomikos, C. A. Demopoulos, I. Zabetakis, *Food Chem.* 100, 560 (2007).

[35] J. Rementzis, S. Antonopoulou, D. Argyropoulos, C. A. Demopoulos, *Adv. Exp. Med. Biol.* 416, 65 (1996).

[36] U. Kaul, S. Sanghvi, V. K. Bahl, V. Dev, H. S. Wasir, *Int. J. Cardiol.* 35, 87 (1992).

[37] F. M. Sacks, P. H. Stone, C. M. Gibson, D. I. Silverman, B. Rosner, R. C. Pasternak, *J. Am. Coll. Cardiol.* 25, 1492 (1995).

[38] "A Study of AMR101 to Evaluate Its Ability to Reduce Cardiovascular Events in High Risk Patients With Hypertriglyceridemia and on Statin. The Primary Objective is to Evaluate the Effect of 4 g/Day AMR101 for Preventing the Occurrence of a First Major Cardiovascular Event. (REDUCE-IT)" http://clinicaltrials.gov/show/NCT01492361.

[39] J. Bosch, H. C. Gerstein, G. R. Dagenais, R. Diaz, L. Dyal, H. Jung, A. P. Maggiono, J. Probstfield, A. Ramachandran, M. C. Riddle, L. E. Ryden, S. Yusuf, *N. Engl. J. Med.* 367, 309 (2013).
[40] W. S. Harris, *Am. J. Clin. Nutr.* 65, 1645S (1997).
[41] J. Geppert, V. Kraft, H. Demmelmair, B. Koletzko, *Br. J. Nutr.* 95, 779 (2006).
[42] D. S. Kelley, D. Siegel, M. Vemuri, B. E. Mackey, *Am. J. Clin. Nutr.* 86, 324 (2007).
[43] C. J. Lavie, R. V. Milani, M. R. Mehra, H. O. Ventura, *J. Am. Coll. Cardiol.* 54, 585 (2009).
[44] W. S. Harris, M. Miller, A. P. Tighe, M. H. Davidson, E. J. Schaefer, *Atherosclerosis* 197, 12 (2008).
[45] M. Borkman, D. J. Chisholm, S. M. Furler, L. H. Storlien, E. W. Kraegen, L. A. Simons, C. N. Chesterman, *Diabetes* 38, 1314 (1989).
[46] B. Vessby, *J. Intern. Med. Suppl.* 731, 207 (1989).
[47] I. L. Mostad, K. S. Bjerve, M. R. Bjorgaas, S. Lydersen, V. Grill, *Am. J. Clin. Nutr.* 84, 540 (2006).
[48] V. M. Montori, A. Farmer, P. C. Wollan, S. F. Dinneen, *Diabetes Care* 23, 1407 (2000).
[49] C. Popp-Snijders, J. A. Schouten, R. J. Heine, J. van der Meer, E. A. van der Veen, *Diabetes Res.* 4, 141 (1987).
[50] J. M. Geleijnse, E. J. Giltay, D. E. Grobbee, A. R. Donders, F. J. Kok, *J. Hypertens.* 20, 1493 (2002).
[51] J. P. Chin, Prostaglandins *Leukot. Essent. Fatty Acids* 50, 211 (1994).
[52] M. B. Engler and M. M. Engler, *Biol. Res. Nurs.* 2, 85 (2000).
[53] H. Shimokawa, J. Y. Lam, J. H. Chesebro, E. J. Bowie, P. M. Vanhoutte, *Circulation* 76, 898 (1987).
[54] S. Grimsgaard, K. H. Bonaa, J. B. Hansen, E. S. Myhre, *Am. J. Clin. Nutr.* 68, 52 (1998).
[55] R. Vandongen, T. A. Mori, V. Burke, L. J. Beilin, J. Morris, J. Ritchie, *Hypertension* 22, 371 (1993).
[56] I. Bairati, L. Roy, F. Meyer, *Can. J. Cardiol.* 8, 41 (1992).
[57] D. Mozaffarian, J. S. Gottdiener, D. S. Siscovick, *Am. J. Cardiol.* 97, 216 (2006).
[58] H. O. Ventura, R. V. Milani, C. J. Lavie, F. W. Smart, D. D. Stapleton, T. S. Toups, H. L. Price, *Circulation* 88, II281(1993).
[59] P. L. McLennan, L. R. Barnden, T. M. Bridle, M. Y. Abeywardena, J. S. Charnock, *Cardiovasc. Res.* 26, 871(1992).

[60] M. Nishimura, A. Nanbu, T. Komori, K. Ohtsuka, H. Takahashi, M. Yoshimura, *Clin. Exp. Pharmacol. Physiol.* 27, 618 (2000).
[61] J. Cabo, R. Alonso, P. Mata, *Br. J. Nutr.* 107, S195 (2012).
[62] M. K. Duda, K. M. O'Shea, W. C. Stanley, *Cardiovasc. Res.* 84, 33 (2009).
[63] P. G. Swann, D. L. Venton, G. C. Le Breton, *FEBS Lett.* 243, 244 (1989).
[64] W. E. Kaminski, E. Jendraschak, R. Kiefl, C. von Schacky, *Blood*, 81, 1871 (1993).
[65] K. Mayer, M. Merfels, M. Muhly-Reinholz, S. Gokorsch, S. Rosseau, J. Lohmeyer, N. Schwarzer, M. Krull, N. Suttorp, F. Grimminger, W. Seeger, *Am. J. Physiol. Heart Circ. Physiol.* 283, H811(2002).
[66] L. G. Gao, J. Cao, Q. X. Mao, X. C. Lu, X. L. Zhou, L. Fan, *Atherosclerosis*, 226, 328 (2013).
[67] P. C. Calder, *Br. J. Clin. Pharmacol.* 75, 645 (2012).
[68] O. D. Rangel-Huerta, C. M. Aguilera, M. D. Mesa, A. Gil, *Br. J. Nutr.* 107, S159 (2012).
[69] L. M. Browning, J. D. Krebs, C. S. Moore, G. D. Mishra, M. A. O'Connell, S. A. Jebb, *Diabetes Obes. Metab.* 9, 70 (2007).
[70] Y. T. Zhao, L. Shao, L. L. Teng, B. Hu, Y. Luo, X. Yu, D. F. Zhang, H. Zhang, *J. Int. Med. Res.* 37, 1831 (2009).
[71] S. K. Raatz, J. T. Silverstein, L. Jahns, M. J. Picklo, *Nutrients* 5, 1081 (2013).
[72] W. Stonehouse, M. R. Pauga, R. Kruger, C. D. Thomson, M. Wong, M. C. Kruger, C, *Br. J. Nutr.* 106, 1231 (2011).
[73] F. Visioli, P. Rise, M. C. Barassi, F. Marangoni, C. Galli, *Lipids* 38 415 (2003).
[74] E. O. Elvevoll, H. Barstad, E. S. Breimo, J. Brox, K. E. Eilertsen, T. Lund, J. O. Olsen, B. Osterud, *Lipids* 41, 1109 (2006).
[75] US Food and Drug Administration, US Environmental Protection Agency (2004) http://www.fda.gov/food/resourcesforyou/consumers/ucm110591.htm.
[76] A. Schecter, P. Cramer, K. Boggess, J. Stanley, O. Papke, J. Olson, A. Silver, M. Schmitz, *J. Toxicol. Environ. Health A.* 63, 1 (2001).
[77] Consumer Lab, https://www.consumerlab.com/reviews/fish_oil_supplements_review/omega3/
[78] T. Tatarczyk, J. Engl, C. Ciardi, M. Laimer, S. Kaser, K. Salzmann, R. Lenners, J. R. Patsch, C. F. Ebenbichler, *Wien Klin. Wochenschr.* 119, 417 (2007).

[79] EFSA Panel on Dietetic Products, *EFSA Journal,* 10, 2815 (2012).
[80] G. L. Russo, *Biochem. Pharmacol.* 77, 937 (2009).
[81] P. Detopoulou and V. Papamikos, *Int. J. Sport Nutr. Exerc. Metab.* in press (2013).
[82] M. Matsuzaki, M. Yokoyama, Y. Saito, H. Origasa, Y. Ishikawa, S. Oikawa, J. Sasaki, H. Hishida, H. Itakura, T. Kita, A. Kitabatake, N. Nakaya, T. Sakata, K. Shimada, K. Shirato, Y. Matsuzawa, *Circ. J.* 73, 1283 (2009).
[83] P. Galan, E. Kesse-Guyot, S. Czernichow, S. Briancon, J. Blacher, S. Hercberg, Effects of B vitamins and omega 3 fatty acids on cardiovascular diseases: a randomised placebo controlled trial, *BMJ*, 341, c6273 (2010).
[84] C. D. Poole, J. P. Halcox, S. Jenkins-Jones, E. S. Carr, M. G. Schifflers, K. K. Ray, C. J. Currie, *Clin. Ther.* 35, 40 (2013).

In: Marine Oils (From Sea to Pharmaceuticals) ISBN: 978-1-63463-747-3
Editor: Ioannis Zabetakis

Chapter 7

Pharmaceutical Applications of Fish Oils

Alexis Garras, David Fraser, Derek Tobin, Runar Vige, and Ida Marie Wold
Pronova BioPharma / BASF, Norway

Abstract

Omega-3 fatty acids have been shown to have an important role in the maintenance of health and treatment of disease since the early observations of health benefits in the Inuit population a few decades ago. Omega-3 fatty acids have since been developed into pharmaceutical products, with high EPA and DHA concentration. Prescription Omega-3 (POM_3) is currently being used for the treatment of post-myocardial infarction and for hypertriglyceridemia, and available safety data support a favourable risk-benefit profile for POM_3. Over the last decades, the mechanisms by which EPA and DHA exert their effect have been partly unveiled. Among others, omega-3 fatty acids reduce TG production in the liver, prevent cardiac arrhythmias through direct effects on ion channels, improve endothelial function, reduce platelet aggregation, and reduce inflammatory burden of atherosclerotic plaques. The production of POM_3 involves complex manufacturing processes, including the removal of environmental toxins and procedures to prevent oxidation. The advent of POM_3 in the early 90s led to the protection of millions of patients from cardiovascular disease.

From the Inuits to POM$_3$

Most of us over the age of 50 who grew up in the Western world remember the gruesome obligatory task of having to ingest an entire soup spoon of cod-liver oil daily. We were told that it was good for us, with no actual rationale; just that it was good for us; fish was good for us and this oil that was produced from cod gave unspecific health benefits, it was a panacea, a snake-oil of some sort. Justification in this belief came from an article from 1979 in which Dyerberg and Bang, two scientists from Denmark, observed an association between the consumption of a high fish and seal diet of Inuits and low rates of myocardial infarction and angina pectoris [1].

These observations in Greenland Eskimo populations demonstrated that despite an almost exclusively fat diet, they rarely suffered from cardiovascular disease, let alone die from it; this finding went against all conventional wisdom at the time. The two scientists then examined the type of fat that the Inuit people consumed (Table 1) [2] with the conclusion that their excellent cardiovascular health was related to the consumption of fish and a high intake of polyunsaturated omega-3 fatty acids.

From that point on several scientists set out to uncover the secrets behind the effects observed by the two Danish pioneers.

In 1989, Burr et al. investigated whether giving dietary advice to patients with a previous myocardial infarction was beneficial [3].

The working theory at the time was that consumption of fatty fish and especially eicosapentanoic acid (EPA) could protect against ischaemic heart disease, in particular in the setting of secondary prevention after a myocardial infarction.

Table 1. Dietary fats in Eskimo and Danish food divided in fat types

Fat types	Eskimos	Danes
Saturated (% of total fatty acids)	22.8	52.7
Monounsaturated (% of total fatty acids)	57.3	34.6
Polyunsaturated (% of total fatty acids)	19.2	12.7
P/S ratio	0.84	0.24
Linolenic class (n-6) (g/day/3000 kcal)	5.4	10.0
Linolenic class (n-3) (g/day/3000 kcal)	13.7	2.8
Monounsaturated, except 16:1 and 18:1 (g/day/3000 kcal)	29.6	2.1

Adapted from [2].

Several observational studies showed that fish consumption was somehow positively associated with ischaemic heart disease [4, 5, 6]. The culprit was saturated fat, while unsaturated fat, especially from fish seemed to show health benefits. Burr and co-workers [3] had men under the age of 70 with a recent myocardial infarction try one of three things: Either 1.) reduce their fat intake to 30% of total calorific intake and increase the polyunsaturated/saturated fatty acid ratio to 1.0, 2.) eat fatty fish portions of 200-400g twice a week consisting of mackerel, herring, kipper, pilchard, sardine, trout or salmon or 3.) increase intake of cereal fibre to 18g per day. What was interesting in the study was that subjects who could not take fish for any reason were instead instructed to take three fish oil capsules that contained 180mg EPA. EPA was the only fatty acid mentioned in the article at the time, but these capsules also contained 120 mg docosahexanoic acid (DHA).

This study was the first controlled investigation of dietary fish intake in the secondary prevention after a myocardial infarction. The results showed that ingestion of fatty fish (or fish oil capsules) reduced mortality by 29%. This observation astounded the authors, but should not have been a surprise especially after the aforementioned Dyerberg and Bang observed similar findings in Norway during and after World War II [7].

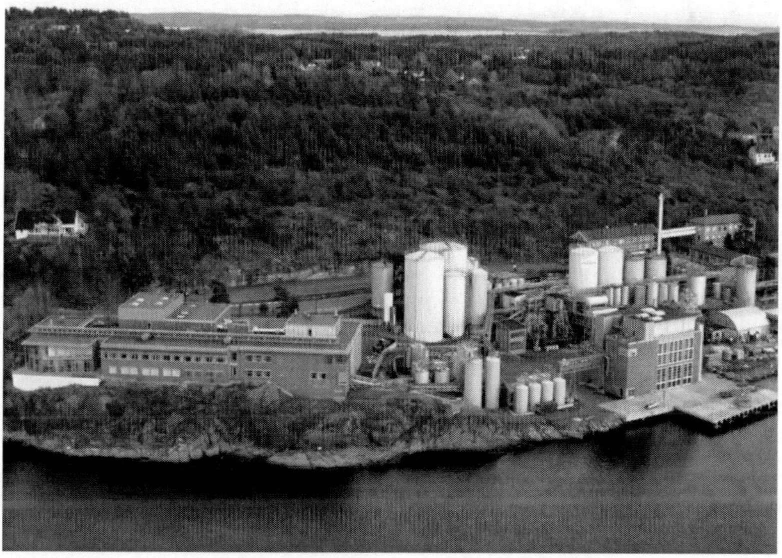

Figure 1. Pronova BioPharma's omega-3 plant in Sandefjord, Norway.

The two Danes observed that at the onset of the war, Norwegians were forced to eat more fish because of food shortages, and mortality due to ischaemic heart disease fell dramatically; it rose again shortly after the war as previous dietary habits were once again resumed. The question following Burr and co-workers' publication was which components of the fish or fish oil were responsible for these observations.

At around the same time a Norwegian company called Pronova was working with fish oil. Pronova's history begins back in 1838 under the name of Johan C. Martens that was first established in the city of Bergen. Martens produced marine oils from fish and one of their first products was cod-liver oil. Pronova and the Italian company Societa Prodotti Antibiotici S.p.A. (SPA) were in the process of refining and concentrating fish oil to a mixture that consisted almost exclusively of EPA and DHA.

In the 80's both companies noticed the effects of high concentrate EPA and DHA on triglycerides in patients with hypertriglyceridemia. Pronova BioPharma was eventually acquired by BASF in 2013. One of the production facilities is pictured in figure 1.

Pharmaceutical Application of Omega-3 to Reduce Plasma Triglycerides and to Prevent Cardiovascular Disease

In the early 90's the significance of lowering lipids such as LDL-cholesterol and triglycerides was sketchy at best. Then in 1994, the importance of lowering LDL-cholesterol was demonstrated in the 4S study [8] where simvastatin was used to lower LDL-cholesterol in patients with coronary artery disease. Lowering of LDL-cholesterol by 35% resulted in 30% reduced risk of dying over the course of the study.

Serious, non-fatal episodes were also substantially lowered by LDL-C reductions. This landmark study heralded a revolution for the treatment of subjects with established heart disease, and all eyes were suddenly on statins.

The early 90's was still a time of confusion as to what the benefits of EPA and DHA were, although the notion of its panacea role was still dominant. However, the established association between cholesterol and cardiovascular morbidity and mortality led to an increased awareness of the role of blood lipids in cardiovascular disease.

The Development of POM_3

Very high levels of triglycerides were known to be a risk factor for the development of pancreatitis. Over the next years more knowledge emerged about the role of triglycerides in cardiovascular disease. It became clearer to the medical community that high blood levels of triglycerides were detrimental for heart health.

Simultaneously, more information was emerging demonstrating that the omega-3 fatty acid ethyl esters that Pronova was producing were able to lower triglycerides in patients with hypertriglyceridemia. The product under development, a refined ethyl ester formulation of fish oil, contained approximately 46% EPA and 38% DHA. In 1994 Omacor®, a pharmaceutical application of a highly concentrated omega-3 product from Pronova was approved as the first POM3 for treatment of hypertriglyceridemia.

Over the next years the pharmaceutical use of omega-3 in treatment of hypertriglyceridemia spread from Norway and Italy, where it all started, to other countries in Europe.

Clinical trials in subjects with hypertriglyceridemia have shown that 4 g/day of POM-3 reduce plasma triglycerides in the range of approximately 25-45%.

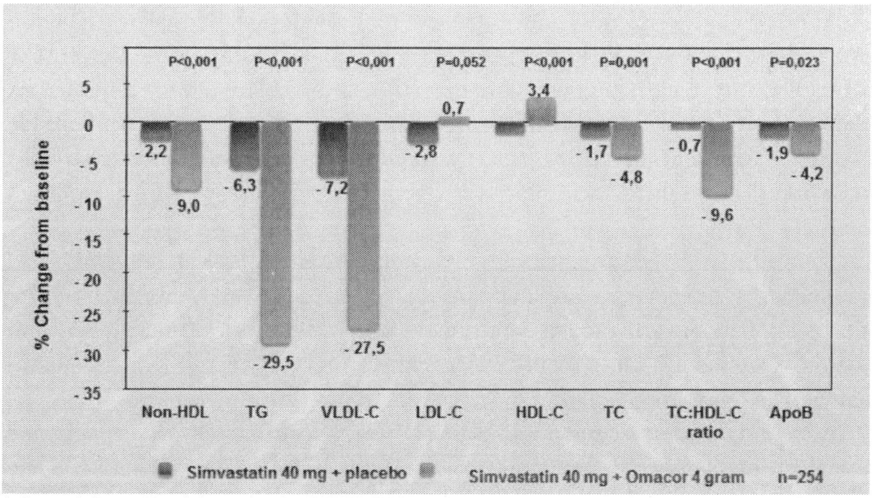

Adapted from Davidson et al. (2007) [10].

Figure 2. Efficacy of POM-3 4 g/day on triglycerides and other lipid markers in statin treated subjects with hypertriglyceridemia.

The COMBOS trial, involving 254 subjects with hypertriglyceridemia already treated with a statin, demonstrated a 29,5% reduction in triglycerides (Figure 2) [9]. The largest reductions, up to 45%, were seen in subjects with very high triglyceride levels (> 5,7 mmol/l, or > 500 mg/dl) [10].

In 1993, the researchers of the Gruppo Italiano per lo Studio della Sopravvivenza nell'Infarto (GISSI) group in Italy had the idea to test the effects of these omega-3 fatty acid ethyl esters in a population similar to the 4S population i.e., subjects who had experienced a myocardial infarction. They grappled with which dose to use in such a population since evidence from the previously mentioned DART study [3] was unable to provide a conclusive efficacious dose. The DART study was based on giving dietary fish advice, or alternatively advising subjects to consume fish oil capsules with quite low omega-3 content. In addition, the omega-3 fatty acids were taken in the form of triglycerides and not ethyl esters as are present in the pharmaceutical product that was under development by Pronova.

The GISSI investigators concluded that they would use one 1-gram capsule per day although most of the data available on the mechanisms of this product had been obtained with much higher, purely pharmacological doses of n-3 PUFA (≥3–4 g/day). The choice of a relatively low-dose regimen (1-g capsule daily) was more acceptable for long-term treatment in a population of patients following Mediterranean dietary habits.

Although the dose was not expected to provide substantial triglyceride lowering effect it was in line with the EPA and DHA intake in the DART study. Over the years it become clear that EPA and DHA could have numerous means of preventing cardiovascular disease other than via its triglyceride lowering effect, and the GISSI group wanted to explore potential mechanisms that worked through the vascular wall or at the cellular level in the injured heart.

The GISSI-Prevenzione trial involved more than 11,000 patients who had experienced a recent myocardial infarction. They were randomly assigned to receive 1-g capsules of omega-3 fatty acid ethyl esters or placebo in addition to usual treatment. All patients were concomitantly treated with standard treatment as recommended after a myocardial infarction.

The study results were published in 1999. No effects were seen in the control group. However, treatment with omega-3 for 3.5 years reduced the number of deaths caused by cardiovascular disease by 30%, and the number of deaths from any cause by 20%. A most striking finding was that the number of sudden deaths was reduced by as much as 45% (figure 3) [11].

Based on the results from the GISSI-Prevenzione trial, POM_3 received approval in 2001 in the European markets for pharmaceutical treatment of patients who had suffered a myocardial infarction (Post-MI), as an adjunct to standard treatment.

Several important milestones were attained over the next years. In 2005 POM_3 was approved in the US for treatment of patients with very high triglyceride levels, and in 2012 POM_3 was approved for treatment of hyperlipidemia in Japan.

As of early 2014 the drug is approved for either hypertriglyceridemia/ hyperlipidemia or post-myocardial infarction, or both, in 61 countries, and in total approximately 2 million patients have been treated with POM_3 worldwide. The product is also known under the brand names Lovaza™, Zodin®, and Lotriga®.

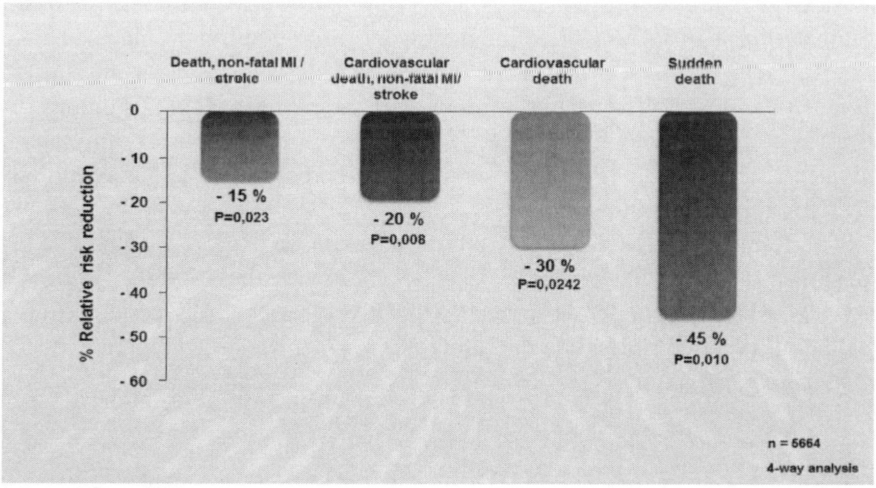

Adapted from [11].

Figure 3. Efficacy of POM-3 1 g/day on mortality and morbidity in the GISSI-Prevenzione trial, 4-way analysis. Relative risk reduction versus control group.

Other Pharmaceutical Omega-3 Products

Epadel®, a refined ethyl ester formulation of fish oil containing mainly EPA, was developed for treatment of hyperlipidemia in Japan as early as 1990. It has since also been approved for treatment of atherosclerosis obliterans.

The JELIS trial investigated the effects of 5 year treatment with Epadel 1800 mg/day in subjects with hypercholesterolaemia. Results showed a 19% reduction in coronary events [12]. The drug is only approved in Japan. Recently a similar high EPA product was developed for treatment of very high triglycerides. Vascepa® was approved in the US in 2012, and is currently not authorized in other markets.

OMEGA-3 IN PREVENTION OF CARDIOVASCULAR AND CARDIOMETABOLIC DISEASE – MECHANISM OF ACTION

The role and mechanisms of omega-3 fatty acids in cardiovascular disease and prevention is probably the most thoroughly studied disease area within omega-3 research. Omega-3 fatty acids are known to influence several cardiovascular risk factors, and thus they work through different mechanisms. Omega-3 fatty acids may alter membrane fluidity and receptor responses through their incorporation into various cell membranes. Direct binding of omega-3 fatty acids to nuclear receptors such as peroxisome proliferator-activated receptor alpha (PPAR-α) and the liver X receptor (LXR) may further directly regulate gene transcription.

The following section will give a brief mechanistic overview of the role of omega-3 fatty acids in various aspects of cardiovascular disease. Omega-3 fatty acids have been demonstrated to positively affect triglyceride levels, endothelial function, inflammation, atherosclerosis, platelet aggregation, heart function and arrhythmias.

Omega-3 Fatty Acids Reduce Plasma Triglycerides through Reducing Both Hepatic TG Secretion and Enhancing Clearance of TG from the Plasma

EPA and DHA reduce triglyceride levels in humans. Harris et al. conducted a pivotal clinical trial in which subjects with very high levels of plasma triglycerides were treated with a 4 gram dose of POM_3.

Results showed that after 4 months of treatment POM_3 intake reduced plasma triglycerides by 45% [10]. Similar results have been demonstrated in other clinical trials with POM_3.

The use of Omega-3 fatty acids in treating hypertriglyceridemia has been nicely summarized in several review papers [13, 14, 15].

Several mechanisms have been suggested for the reduction of triglycerides (figure 4). These include 1) decreased hepatic lipogenesis through a decreased conversion of acetyl-CoA to fatty acids; 2) increased β-oxidation of free fatty acids; 3) the inhibition of phosphatidic acid phosphatase and diacylglycerol acyltransferase (both enzymes that catalyse important steps in triglyceride synthesis); 4) potential increased degradation of apolipoprotein B; and 5) increased activity of lipoprotein lipase, an enzyme that increases the conversion of VLDL particles to LDL particles. In essence, treatment with omega-3 fatty acids reduce the availability of fatty acids for triglyceride synthesis in the liver, and increase the breakdown and removal of triglycerides in the circulating VLDL particles and chylomicrons. The result is lower triglyceride levels in the blood.

How the aforementioned observations are effectuated may be explained at the gene transcriptional level. Nuclear receptors such as the liver X receptor, hepatocyte nuclear factor–4α (HNF-4α), farnesol X receptor, and peroxisome proliferator–activated receptors (PPARs) are each regulated by sterol receptor element binding protein–1c (SREBP-1c), the main genetic switch controlling lipogenesis. EPA and DHA inhibit hepatic lipogenesis by reducing levels of SREBP-1c, up-regulating fatty oxidation in the liver and skeletal muscle through activation of PPAR, and enhancing flux of glucose to glycogen through down-regulation of HNF-4α. The results of this co-ordination are to direct fatty acids from triglyceride storage toward oxidation, thereby reducing the substrate available for very-low-density lipoprotein (VLDL) synthesis.

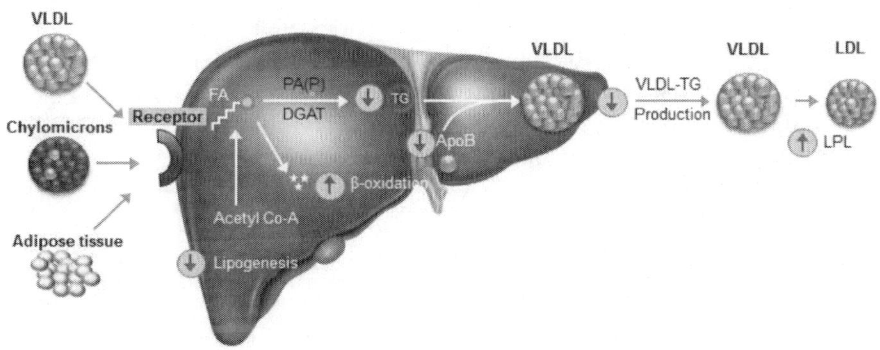

Figure 4. Mechanisms by which EPA and DHA are believed to reduce plasma triglycerides.

Another suggested mechanism is that EPA and DHA undergo extensive peroxidation, which stimulates the degradation of apolipoprotein B, resulting in the reduction of VLDL secretion from the liver [16].

Omega-3 Fatty Acids Reduce Sudden Cardiac Death by Preventing Ventricular Rhythm Disturbances

One of the most interesting observations in the GISSI-Prevenzione study was the reduction of sudden death by 45% (55 patients died in the POM_3 group versus 99 patients in the control group) in patients who received 1 gram prescription omega-3 ethyl esters. Sudden deaths are typically in the form of heart rhythm disturbances and cardiac arrest. This effect accounted for the major part of the reduction seen in total mortality in the GISSI-Prevenzione trial [11].

A possible mechanism of action has subsequently been explained [17]. In the normal functioning heart, the depolarization and repolarization of myocytes provides the regular, rhythmic contractions during a heartbeat. This cycle is well regulated and involves an influx and efflux of various ions, such as sodium, calcium and potassium. The right balance of these ions is a prerequisite to the normo-rhythmia of the heart. Sodium ions enter myocytes via sodium channels that are defined as "rapid sodium ion channels". In other words, influx to the cells occurs in spurts and not as a continuum. Influx of ions in this manner commences the depolarization process and is followed by an influx of calcium ions which causes the myocytes to contract. Thereafter, the process of repolarization begins and the cycle is completed by a rebalancing of electrolytes. In the ischaemic heart, the rapid sodium channels are defunct and there is a continuous leakage of sodium ions into the myocyte (figure 5). This causes more calcium ions to enter the cells giving a surplus of intracellular calcium. Too much intracellular calcium inevitably leads to an increased incidence of ventricular arrhythmias.

The effects of EPA and DHA have been attributed to the incorporation of free fatty acids into the microenvironment of ion channels and the ensuing conformational change. This hypothesis has been tested in cell models and in various animal models. In a series of experiments (reviewed by Leaf et al. [18]) it was shown that EPA and DHA inhibit Na+ channel activity. In another study, administration of omega-3 fatty acids were demonstrated to prevent fatal ventricular arrhythmias in dogs who had undergone a recent surgically induced myocardial infarction [19].

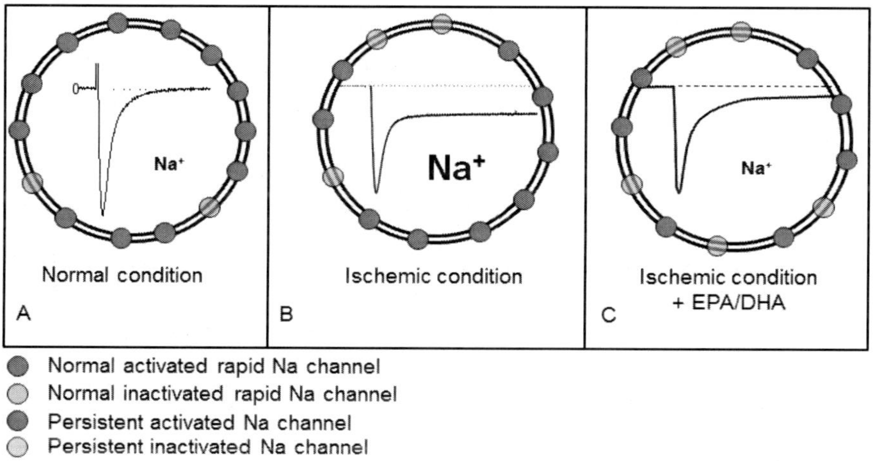

Figure 5. Sodium channels in the normal versus the ischemic myocyte and the effects of EPA and DHA; (A) illustrates the action potential return to baseline in the normal non-ischemic condition. The dark blue circles represent normal activated rapid sodium channels, while the light blue circles represent normal inactivated sodium channels. Panel (B) shows the situation in the ischemic condition whereby the influx of sodium ions is greater than the normal condition; this is due to the presence of persistent activated sodium channels (red circles). The orange circles represent persistent inactivated sodium channels. (C) illustrates the effects of EPA and DHA on the ischemic condition; it seems as if the activity of several rapid sodium channels is restored, thereby reducing the levels of intracellular calcium, bringing the action potential almost back to normal and therefore leading to less arrhythmias.

Although both EPA and DHA are active in this respect, some findings indicate that DHA is superior to EPA in restoring normal rhythm [17] (Figure 6).DONE TO HERE

Interestingly, the reductions in sudden death in the GISSI-Prevenzione trial [11] were closely linked to subjects with impaired pump function of the heart, referred to as heart failure. These findings were hypothesis-generating for designing the GISSI-Heart Failure trial (GISSI-HF).

Approximately 7000 patients with heart failure were randomly allocated to treatment with prescription omega-3 fatty acids, or placebo.

Results showed that 3,9 years of treatment with 1g omega-3 fatty acids reduced the incidence of death with 9% and the combination of death and hospitalization for cardiovascular reasons by 8%.

These findings were mainly related to reduction of cardiac rhythm disturbances [20], and thus confirmed the previous hypothesis.

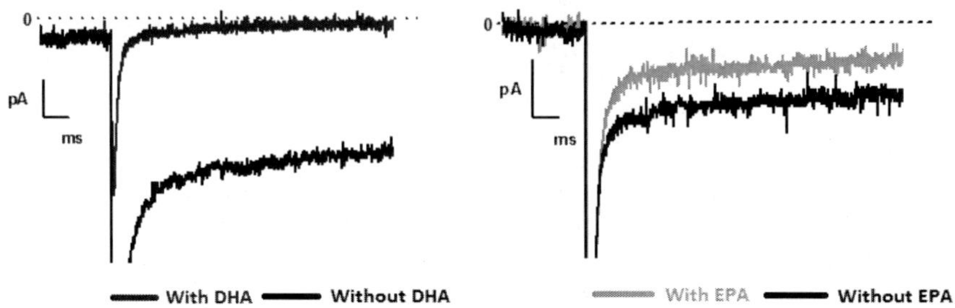

Figure 6. Concentration-response curves on late sodium current. Typical effect of acute application of DHA and EPA results in blockage of veratridine-induced late sodium current.

Omega-3 Fatty Acids Improve Cardiac Function by Enhancing the Contractile Function of the Cardiac Cells

Omega-3 fatty acids are also believed to have other mechanistic effects on the cells of the heart. In the GISSI-HF trial treatment with omega-3 fatty acids was also shown to increase the pump function of the heart, measured as "left ventricular ejection fraction" [21]. A small clinical study demonstrated that treatment of patients with severe heart failure of non-ischemic origin with prescription omega-3 fatty acids 1g /day or 4g /day for three months significantly improved the pump function of the heart, measured as "left ventricular ejection fraction [22]. A similar study showed that treatment with prescription omega-3 fatty acids for 12 months significantly increased ejection fraction in patients with a dilated heart and impaired pump function [23].

Together these studies suggest that omega-3 fatty acids improve contractile properties of the cells of the heart by reducing circulating levels of cytokines, improving efficiency of ATP generation and thus mechanical efficiency, reversed dysfunction of the endothelium, and increased respiratory efficiency of the heart muscle.

Omega-3 Fatty Acids Decrease Platelet Aggregation by Inhibiting Synthesis of Arachidonic Acid

Platelet aggregation is carefully regulated by the metabolites of arachidonic acid.

Thromboxane A2, a metabolite of arachidonic acid, stimulates platelet aggregation. On the other hand, arachidonic acid derived prostacyclin is a vasodilator and opposes platelet aggregation. Omega-3 acts as a competitive substrate to omega-6 which undergoes metabolism to arachidonic acid. Omega-3 metabolites have a reduced inflammatory activity and lower platelet aggregation potential compared to omega-6 derived eicosanoids [24].

Consequently, insufficient intake of omega-3 fatty acids may disrupt the omega-3:omega-6 balance and contribute to a pro-inflammatory and pro-atherogenic state. The net result of higher tissue levels of omega-3 fatty acids is thus antithrombotic. In a clinical trial, prescription omega-3 fatty acids reduced platelet activity biomarkers in subjects with coronary artery disease and hypertriglyceridemia [25].

Omega-3 Fatty Acids Stabilize Atherosclerotic Plaque by Reducing the Grade of Inflammation and Altering Factors Involved in Fibrous Cap Formation

Lipoproteins circulating in the blood, such as LDL and VLDL, carry large amounts of cholesterol and other lipids. Lipoproteins stick to adhesion molecules that are expressed in the endothelial cell linings of the vascular wall. The formation of an atherosclerotic plaque is directly related to migration of atherogenic lipoproteins into the atheroma, with subsequent oxidation of the lipoproteins, and lipid deposition. The build-up of atheromatous plaque is a slow process, developed over a period of several years through a complex series of cellular events occurring within the arterial wall. This process is closely linked to inflammatory processes in which macrophages, as part of the body's defence system, enter the sub-endothelial space to deal with the foreign body. The macrophages engulf the lipids and form foam cells that are deposited within the arterial wall. The result is the formation of atheroma and atherosclerotic plaque covering the deposit.

It has been demonstrated that atherosclerotic plaques from patients treated with omega-3 fatty acids are less heavily infiltrated with macrophages than those treated with placebo [26]. EPA content of the plaque phospholipids have been shown to be inversely associated with plaque instability and plaque inflammation. Moreover prescription omega-3 fatty acids were demonstrated to reduce the expression of certain matrix metalloproteinases, certain cytokines and intracellular adhesion molecules in plaques [27].

Together these findings indicate that omega-3 fatty acids can thicken the fibrous cap covering the plaques, thereby making them more stable and less prone to rupture.

Omega-3 Fatty Acids Reduce Blood Pressure and Heart Rate through Improvements in Endothelial Function

A meta-analysis involving 36 randomized trials showed that dietary supplementation with omega-3 provided moderate, but statistically significant, reductions in systolic and diastolic blood pressure [28].

Furthermore, in one study treatment with prescription omega-3 fatty acids 4 g/day for four months reduced mean systolic and diastolic blood pressure by 6 mm Hg and 5 mm Hg respectively [29].

Two main mechanisms have been suggested to explain this effect. Incorporation of omega-3 fatty acids into membrane phospholipids is believed to increase systemic arterial compliance [30]. EPA and DHA has also been shown to improve endothelial function, a finding which is consistent with the observation that the blood pressure lowering effects of omega-3 fatty acids is greater in populations with arterial stiffness and microvascular dysfunction, such as hypertensive and older populations. The effect is believed to be mediated through four possible mechanisms: 1) suppression of thromboxane A_2 or cyclic endoperoxides; 2) increased endothelial synthesis of nitric oxide (NO); 3) improvement of vascular smooth muscle cell sensitivity to NO; and 4) decreased formation of reactive oxygen species. Prescription omega-3 fatty acids have been shown to increase the elasticity of the arteries in obese subjects [31], and improve endothelial function in subjects with type II diabetes in the postprandial state [32]. A meta-analysis further found that intake of omega-3 fatty acids can significantly reduce heart rate [33].

The Active Pharmaceutical Ingredient (API) in Omacor® Is Made from an Eight Step Purification Process

The manufacturing of the Omacor® API is an eight step process that is outlined in Figure 7.

The starting point for the manufacturing process is crude fish oil. Crude oil consists of a mixture of saturated and unsaturated fat in the form of triglycerides and free fatty acids from fish such as sardines and mackerel.

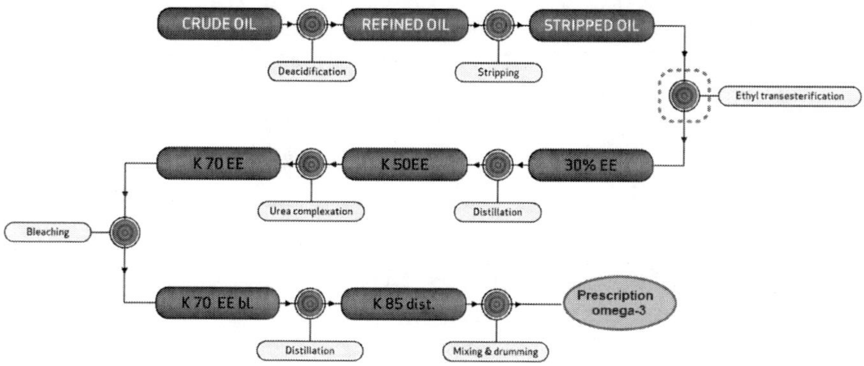

Figure 7. Schematic representation of the process of manufacturing of the API in Omacor®.

In addition, the crude oil naturally comprises cholesterol, vitamins (vitamin A, D) and a number of environmental pollutants. There is significant variability in the types and levels of persistant organic pollutants (POPs) depending on the source of the fish oil [34]. The concentration of EPA and DHA in the crude oil is typically 18% and 12%, respectively.

The first step in the manufacturing of the Omacor® API is de-acidification in which free fatty acids are removed. Next is the patented step of stripping the oil. This step removes cholesterol, environmental pollutants and vitamins. Thereafter comes a transesterification step where the triglycerides are mixed with ethanol and sodium ethylate and converted to ethyl esters and glycerol. The next step involves distillation that leads to a more concentrated mixture of EPA and DHA, followed by a urea complexation step that removes the more saturated fatty acids. The oil is then bleached to remove oxidation products and then further distilled to get to the final concentration of 84% EPA and DHA (480 mg EPA and 360 mg DHA per 1000 mg of oil), followed by mixing and drumming of the final product.

Figure 8 shows the oil at various steps during the manufacturing process: from dark, crude fish oil to the highly concentrated prescription omega-3 which is completely clear.

From the site of manufacturing, the oil is transferred to encapsulators either on the European mainland or in the US, where soft gelatin capsules are produced, tested and subsequently released to the markets.

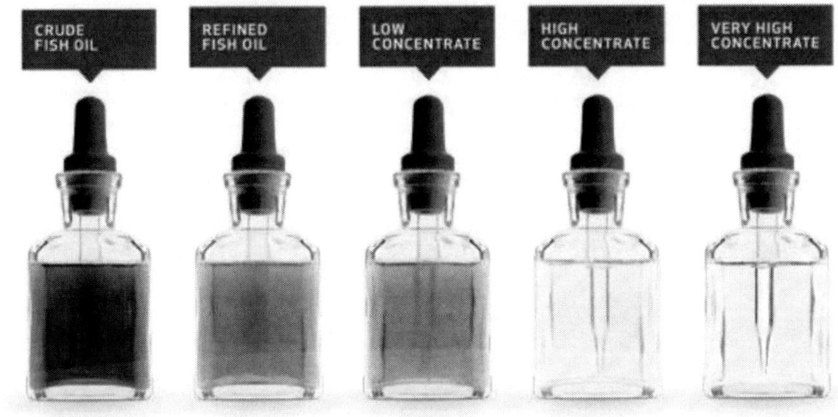

Figure 8. Appearance of fish oil at various stages of the prescription omega-3 manufacturing process. Crude fish oil (far left) is dark brown, while the final active pharmaceutical ingredient (far right) is completely clear.

POM$_3$ Has a Favourable Risk-Benefit Profile

Omacor® is currently approved in 85 countries worldwide. In most markets, the trademark used is Omacor®, but the product in some markets is known under the trademarks Lovaza (US only), Zodin, or Lotriga (Japan only). The approved indications are 1) Post Myocardical Infarction (Post-MI); and 2) Hypertriglyceridemia (HTG). The two indications are based on different mechanisms of action as outlined earlier, and differ with regards to dosing. For Post-MI treatment the dose is 1 g/day and for HTG the dose is 2-4 g/day. Since its introduction in 1994 it has been estimated that cumulative patient exposure is more than 7.5 million patient years.

Omacor® is considered to have a favourable safety profile. Although adverse reactions occur, they are mostly mild and reversible. Most common adverse drug reactions include gastrointestinal disturbances such as fishy burps, distension, diarrhoea, and flatulence [35].

Some published studies with omega-3 fatty acids have demonstrated a moderate increase in bleeding time. However bleeding time has not exceeded normal limits. Nevertheless, patients receiving anticoagulant therapy should be monitored and the dosage of anticoagulant adjusted if necessary. The US label for Lovaza is based on subjects with triglycerides > 500 mg/dl (> 5,7 mmol/l), Table 2 [36].

Table 2. Adverse events in randomized, placebo-controlled, double-blind, parallel group studies for very high TG Levels (>500 mg/dL) that used Lovaza 4g/day

BODY SYSTEM Adverse Event	LOVAZA (N = 226)		Placebo (N = 228)	
	n	%	n	%
Subjects with at least 1 adverse event	80	35.4	63	27.6
Body as a whole				
Back pain	5	2.2	3	1.3
Flu syndrome	8	3.5	3	1.3
Infection	10	4.4	5	2.2
Pain	4	1.8	3	1.3
Cardiovascular				
Angina pectoris	3	1.3	2	0.9
Digestive				
Dyspepsia	7	3.1	6	2.6
Eructation	11	4.9	5	2.2
Skin				
Rash	4	1.8	1	0.4
Special senses				
Taste perversion	6	2.7	0	0.0

Adapted from [36].

POM_3 containing pure EPA has a similar safety profile to Omacor®. Post marketing experience with EPA products for the treatment of very high triglycerides is however more limited than for Omacor®.

Overall, available safety data support a favourable risk-benefit profile for POM_3.

The Difference between POM_3 and Supplements

Fish oil as defined by European Pharmacopoeia usually contains approximately 30% of the fatty acids EPA and DHA of which EPA is 18% and DHA 12%; in other words, a capsule containing a total of 1000 mg oil would contain approximately 180 mg EPA and 120 mg DHA in the form of triglycerides. This implies 70% of other substances and some of these are shown in the chromatogram displayed in figure 9.

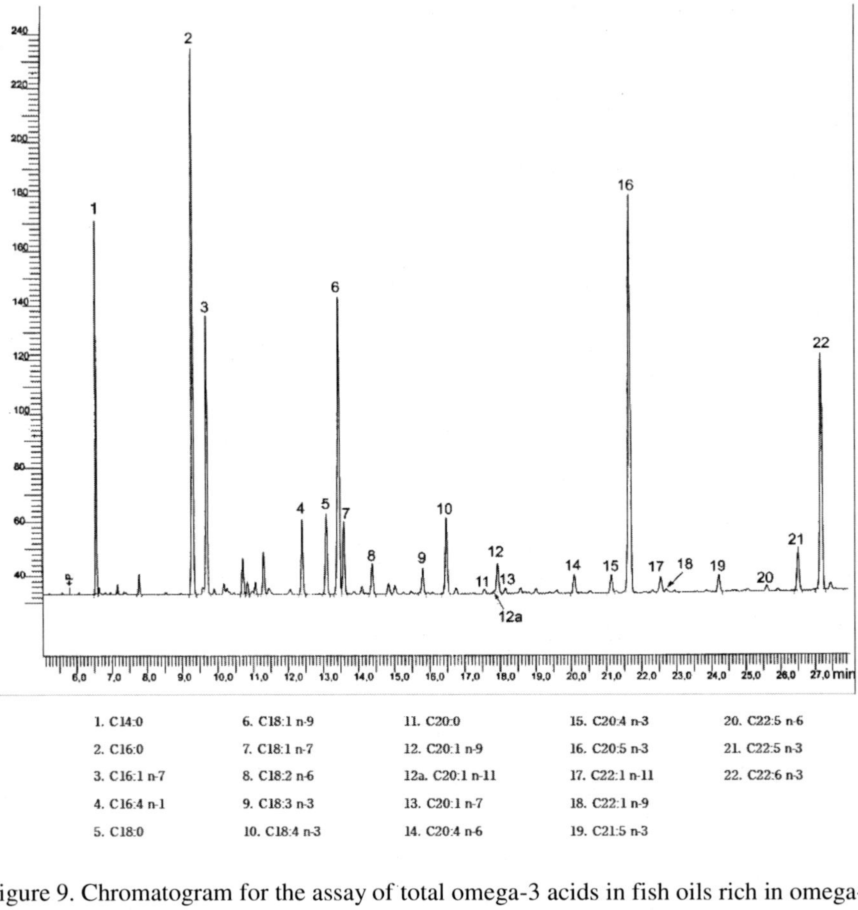

1. C14:0	6. C18:1 n-9	11. C20:0	15. C20:4 n-3	20. C22:5 n-6
2. C16:0	7. C18:1 n-7	12. C20:1 n-9	16. C20:5 n-3	21. C22:5 n-3
3. C16:1 n-7	8. C18:2 n-6	12a. C20:1 n-11	17. C22:1 n-11	22. C22:6 n-3
4. C16:4 n-1	9. C18:3 n-3	13. C20:1 n-7	18. C22:1 n-9	
5. C18:0	10. C18:4 n-3	14. C20:4 n-6	19. C21:5 n-3	

Figure 9. Chromatogram for the assay of total omega-3 acids in fish oils rich in omega-3 acids [37].

These other substances include saturated fatty acids, cholesterol, oxidation products, and a number of environmental pollutants.

The environmental pollutants include man-made chemical substances referred to as persistent organic pollutants (POPs). POPs is a collective term including polychlorinated biphenyls (both dioxin-like and non-dioxin-like), dioxins, dichlorodiphenyltrichloroethane (DDT) and brominated flame retardants. The common features for the POPs is that they are lipophilic substances that accumulate throughout the food chain, have a very long half-life and are found across large geographical areas. The lipophilic nature and the persistency of these substances result in bioaccumulation.

Table 3. Sum of PCBs and TEQs measured in fish oils around the world. Dioxin-like PCBs constitute 60-90% of the TEQ value [38-41]

Component	Country	TEQ pg/g	Sum PCBs ng/g	References
Salmon oil	Canada	70.1	36-105	Bourdon et al., 2010
Salmon oil	Canada	18.0	36-170	Rawn et al., 2009
Cod liver oil	UK	12.9-46.0	153	Fernandes et al., 2006
Cod liver oil	Spain	9.4-14.5	49.7-98.3	Marti et al., 2010
Cod liver oil	Ireland	0.6-37.6		Marti et al., 2010
Fish oil	Japan	1.3-29.5		Marti et al., 2010

Many fish oil supplements on the market contain very high concentrations of POPs, as shown in table 3.

Adverse health effects such as metabolic disorders, neurodevelopmental disorders and cancer have been closely associated to exposure to POPs [42]. Increased concentrations of environmental pollutants may also increase the incidence of cardiovascular disease [43]. Humans are inevitably exposed to POPs through food and to some extent air and drinking water.

To keep the overall concentration below the safe limits set by health authorities such as the World Health Organisation (WHO) and the European Union (EU) [44] and thereby reduce the risk of adverse effects, it is important that omega-3 products are highly purified.

Ethyl Esters Versus Triglycerides: Different Intestinal Absorption Rates of EPA and DHA

Much has been made of the different absorption between triglyceride and ethyl ester omega-3 preparations. Whether an EPA and DHA level required for a given biological activity is reached depends not only on the fatty acid release from fatty acid stores but also on the absorption of orally administered EPA and DHA. The type of ester bond of EPA and DHA has consequences for the absorption kinetics of EPA and DHA and consequently duodenal uptake rates differ between triglycerides and ethyl esters.

Triglycerides are rapidly degraded by pancreatic lipase and, in the case of polyunsaturated fatty acids, particularly by carboxyl ester hydrolase.

Absorbed lipids are passed on to the lymphatic system and transported to the circulation via the thoracic duct, thereby bypassing the liver. After entering the blood circulation they reach the heart where they are hydrolyzed by lipoprotein lipase into fatty acids and taken up into cardiomyocytes. In addition to being integrated in the cell membrane, 80% of metabolic energy consumption of the heart is derived from fatty acids. Therefore, EPA and DHA levels measured in the lymph are of interest when assessing therapeutic profiles of various omega-3 preparations.

Synthetic ethyl esters of EPA and DHA are absorbed more slowly than triglycerides. In a study by Ikeda et al. EPA and DHA either as triglycerides or as ethyl esters were administered to rats, and the recovery of EPA and DHA was determined in the lymph at various time points [45].

Within 3 hours after administration, the recovery in the lymph of the respective fatty acids was higher in the case of triglycerides compared to ethyl esters. However, the 9-24 hour recovery of EPA and DHA in the forms of ethyl esters was approximately doubled compared to that of triglycerides, and total EPA and DHA recovery within 24 hours did not differ between ethyl esters and triglycerides.

One of the consequences is that the EPA and DHA supply to the circulation is maintained at a higher level in the second half of a 24 h period which is of importance, since ventricular tachyarrhythmias are more abundant in the early morning hours [46]. Lymph EPA and DHA levels arising from fish consumption during the preceding day would thus be expected to be lower than in the case of an ethyl ester administration.

The different absorption kinetics seen in the rat appears to also apply to humans. The recovery of EPA in the blood was lower within an 8 h period when compared with triglycerides [47], while there was essentially no difference in the long-term plasma concentration of EPA and DHA involvingtime periods up to 28 days [48].

In summary, there is convincing evidence that ethyl esters result in a delayed intestinal uptake of EPA and DHA the first hours after intake. However in the long-term, steady state levels are similar between ethyl ester and triglycerides. An ethyl ester preparation has the advantage of providing 840 mg EPA and DHA in 1 g capsule, whereby the retarded absorption is associated with a sustained delivery of EPA and DHA to target organs such as the heart. Of particular importance is that long-chain fatty acids including EPA and DHA are transported in the lymph and after intestinal absorption reach the heart before their level can be adjusted by the liver.

REFERENCES

[1] Dyerberg, J. and H. O. Bang, Haemostatic function and platelet polyunsaturated fatty acids in Eskimos. *Lancet*, 1979. 2(8140): p. 433-5.

[2] Bang, H. O., J. Dyerberg and H. M. Sinclair, The composition of the Eskimo food in north western Greenland. *Am. J. Clin. Nutr.*, 1980. 33 (12): p. 2657-61.

[3] Burr, M. L., et al., Effects of changes in fat, fish, and fibre intakes on death and myocardial reinfarction: diet and reinfarction trial (DART). *Lancet*, 1989. 2(8666): p. 757-61.

[4] Kromhout, D., E. B. Bosschieter and C. de Lezenne Coulander, The inverse relation between fish consumption and 20-year mortality from coronary heart disease. *N. Engl. J. Med.*, 1985. 312(19): p. 1205-9.

[5] Fish consumption and mortality from coronary heart disease. *N. Engl. J. Med.*, 1985. 313(13): p. 820-4.

[6] Norell, S. E., et al., Fish consumption and mortality from coronary heart disease. *Br. Med. J.* (Clin. Res. Ed.), 1986. 293(6544): p. 426.

[7] Bang, H. O. and J. Dyerberg, Personal reflections on the incidence of ischaemic heart disease in Oslo during the Second World War. *Acta Med. Scand.,* 1981. 210(4): p. 245-8.

[8] Kjekshus, J. and T. R. Pedersen, Reducing the risk of coronary events: evidence from the Scandinavian Simvastatin Survival Study (4S). *Am. J. Cardiol.,* 1995. 76(9): p. 64C-68C.

[9] Davidson, M. H., et al., Efficacy and tolerability of adding prescription omega-3 fatty acids 4 g/d to simvastatin 40 mg/d in hypertriglyceridemic patients: an 8-week, randomized, double-blind, placebo-controlled study. *Clin. Ther.*, 2007. 29(7): p. 1354-67.

[10] Harris, W. S., et al., Safety and efficacy of Omacor in severe hypertriglyceridemia. *J. Cardiovasc. Risk*, 1997. 4(5-6): p. 385-91.

[11] GISSI-PrevenzioneInvestigators, Dietary supplementation with n-3 polyunsaturated fatty acids and vitamin E after myocardial infarction: results of the GISSI-Prevenzione trial. Gruppo Italiano per lo Studio della Sopravvivenza nell'Infarto miocardico. *Lancet*, 1999. 354(9177): p. 447-55.

[12] Yokoyama, M., et al., Effects of eicosapentaenoic acid on major coronary events in hypercholesterolaemic patients (JELIS): a randomised open-label, blinded endpoint analysis. *Lancet*, 2007. 369 (9567): p. 1090-8.

[13] Bays, H., Clinical overview of Omacor: a concentrated formulation of omega-3 polyunsaturated fatty acids. *Am. J. Cardiol.*, 2006. 98(4A): p. 71i-76i.

[14] Skulas-Ray, A. C., et al., Omega-3 fatty acid concentrates in the treatment of moderate hypertriglyceridemia. *Expert Opin. Pharmacother.*, 2008. 9(7): p. 1237-48.

[15] Lewis, A., et al., Treatment of hypertriglyceridemia with omega-3 fatty acids: a systematic review. *J. Am. Acad. Nurse Pract.*, 2004. 16(9): p. 384-95.

[16] Davidson, M. H., Mechanisms for the hypotriglyceridemic effect of marine omega-3 fatty acids. *Am. J. Cardiol.*, 2006. 98(4A): p. 27i-33i.

[17] Pignier, C., et al., Direct protective effects of poly-unsaturated fatty acids, DHA and EPA, against activation of cardiac late sodium current: a mechanism for ischemia selectivity. *Basic Res. Cardiol.*, 2007. 102(6): p. 553-64.

[18] Leaf, A., et al., Clinical prevention of sudden cardiac death by n-3 polyunsaturated fatty acids and mechanism of prevention of arrhythmias by n-3 fish oils. *Circulation*, 2003. 107(21): p. 2646-52.

[19] Billman, G. E., J. X. Kang and A. Leaf, Prevention of sudden cardiac death by dietary pure omega-3 polyunsaturated fatty acids in dogs. *Circulation*, 1999. 99(18): p. 2452-7.

[20] Gissi, H. F. I., et al., Effect of n-3 polyunsaturated fatty acids in patients with chronic heart failure (the GISSI-HF trial): a randomised, double-blind, placebo-controlled trial. *Lancet*, 2008. 372(9645): p. 1223-30.

[21] Ghio, S., et al., Effects of n-3 polyunsaturated fatty acids and of rosuvastatin on left ventricular function in chronic heart failure: a substudy of GISSI-HF trial. *Eur. J. Heart Fail.*, 2010. 12(12): p. 1345-53.

[22] Moertl, D., et al., Dose-dependent effects of omega-3-polyunsaturated fatty acids on systolic left ventricular function, endothelial function, and markers of inflammation in chronic heart failure of nonischemic origin A double-blind, placebo-controlled, 3-arm study. *Am. Heart J.,* 2011. 161(5): p. 915 e1-9.

[23] Nodari, S., et al., Effects of n-3 polyunsaturated fatty acids on left ventricular function and functional capacity in patients with dilated cardiomyopathy. *J. Am. Coll. Cardiol.*, 2011. 57(7): p. 870-9.

[24] Calder, P. C., n-3 Fatty acids and cardiovascular disease: evidence explained and mechanisms explored. *Clin. Sci.* (Lond.), 2004. 107(1): p. 1-11.

[25] Serebruany, V. L., *Early Impact of Prescription Omega-3 Fatty Acids on Platelet Biomarkers in Patients with Coronary Artery Disease and Hypertriglyceridemia.* 2011.

[26] Thies, F., et al., Association of n-3 polyunsaturated fatty acids with stability of atherosclerotic plaques: a randomised controlled trial. *Lancet,* 2003. 361(9356): p. 477-85.

[27] Cawood, A. L., et al., Eicosapentaenoic acid (EPA) from highly concentrated n-3 fatty acid ethyl esters is incorporated into advanced atherosclerotic plaques and higher plaque EPA is associated with decreased plaque inflammation and increased stability. *Atherosclerosis,* 2010. 212(1): p. 252-9.

[28] Geleijnse, J. M., et al., Blood pressure response to fish oil supplementation: metaregression analysis of randomized trials. *J. Hypertens.,* 2002. 20(8): p. 1493-9.

[29] Prisco, D., et al., Effect of medium-term supplementation with a moderate dose of n-3 polyunsaturated fatty acids on blood pressure in mild hypertensive patients. *Thromb. Res.,* 1998. 91(3): p. 105-12.

[30] Nestel, P., et al., The n-3 fatty acids eicosapentaenoic acid and docosahexaenoic acid increase systemic arterial compliance in humans. *Am. J. Clin. Nutr.,* 2002. 76(2): p. 326-30.

[31] Wong, A. T., et al., Supplementation with n3 fatty acid ethyl esters increases large and small artery elasticity in obese adults on a weight loss diet. *J. Nutr.,* 2013. 143(4): p. 437-41.

[32] Stirban, A., et al., Effects of n-3 fatty acids on macro- and microvascular function in subjects with type 2 diabetes mellitus. *Am. J. Clin. Nutr.,* 2010. 91(3): p. 808-13.

[33] Mozaffarian, D., et al., Effect of fish oil on heart rate in humans: a meta-analysis of randomized controlled trials. *Circulation,* 2005. 112(13): p. 1945-52.

[34] Jacobs, M. N., A. Covaci and P. Schepens, Investigation of selected persistent organic pollutants in farmed Atlantic salmon (Salmo salar), salmon aquaculture feed, and fish oil components of the feed. *Environ. Sci. Technol.,* 2002. 36(13): p. 2797-805.

[35] *Omacor Summary of Product Characteristics.* http://www.medicines.org.uk/emc/medicine/10312/indications.

[36] *Lovaza Package Insert.* http://www.accessdata.fda.gov/drugsatfda_docs/label/2009/021654s023lbl.pdf.

[37] Pronova-BioPharma, *Data on File.* 2014.

[38] Bourdon, J. A., et al., Polychlorinated biphenyls (PCBs) contamination and aryl hydrocarbon receptor (AhR) agonist activity of Omega-3 polyunsaturated fatty acid supplements: implications for daily intake of dioxins and PCBs. *Food Chem. Toxicol.*, 2010. 48(11): p. 3093-7.

[39] Rawn, D. F., et al., Persistent organic pollutants in fish oil supplements on the Canadian market: polychlorinated biphenyls and organochlorine insecticides. *J. Food Sci.*, 2009. 74(1): p. T14-9.

[40] Fernandes, A. R., et al., Dioxins and polychlorinated biphenyls (PCBs) in fish oil dietary supplements: occurrence and human exposure in the UK. *Food Addit. Contam.*, 2006. 23(9): p. 939-47.

[41] Marti, M., et al., Persistent organic pollutants (PCDD/Fs, dioxin-like PCBs, marker PCBs, and PBDEs) in health supplements on the Spanish market. *Chemosphere*, 2010. 78(10): p. 1256-62.

[42] Mrema, E. J., et al., Persistent organochlorinated pesticides and mechanisms of their toxicity. *Toxicology*, 2013. 307: p. 74-88.

[43] Aminov, Z., et al., Analysis of the effects of exposure to polychlorinated biphenyls and chlorinated pesticides on serum lipid levels in residents of Anniston, Alabama. *Environ. Health*, 2013. 12: p. 108.

[44] Gies, A., et al., Risk assessment of dioxins and dioxin-like PCBs in food--comments by the German Federal Environmental Agency. *Chemosphere*, 2007. 67(9): p. S344-9.

[45] Ikeda, I., et al., Lymphatic transport of eicosapentaenoic and docosahexaenoic acids as triglyceride, ethyl ester and free acid, and their effect on cholesterol transport in rats. *Life Sci.*, 1993. 52(16): p. 1371-9.

[46] Kozak, M., L. Krivan and B. Semrad, Circadian variations in the occurrence of ventricular tachyarrhythmias in patients with implantable cardioverter defibrillators. *Pacing Clin. Electrophysiol.*, 2003. 26(3): p. 731-5.

[47] Lawson, L. D. and B. G. Hughes, Human absorption of fish oil fatty acids as triacylglycerols, free acids, or ethyl esters. *Biochem. Biophys. Res. Commun.*, 1988. 152(1): p. 328-35.

[48] Luley, C., H. Wieland and J. Grünwald, Bioavailability of Omega-3 fatty acids: ethyl ester preparations are as suitable as triglyceride preparations. *Akt. Ernær Med.*, 1990. 15: p. 123-125.

In: Marine Oils (From Sea to Pharmaceuticals) ISBN: 978-1-63463-747-3
Editor: Ioannis Zabetakis

Chapter 8

IS FISH SOMETHING MORE THAN MARINE OILS?

Ioannis Zabetakis

Laboratory of Food Chemistry, Faculty of Chemistry, School of Sciences, National and Kapodistrian University of Athens, Athens, Greece

ABSTRACT

In light of growing evidence that the supplementation of omega-3 PUFAs does not have a positive effect on CVDs, a novel approach is suggested. Fish could be fed with compounds that have been proved beneficial against CVDs (e.g., olive industry by-products) and novel nutraceuticals could be derived from those novel aquacultured fish species. Some suggestions for novel applications are presented.

TO OMEGA-3 OR NOT TO OMEGA-3?

Today, there is considerable controversy regarding the association of omega-3 polyunsaturated fatty acids (PUFAs) and cardiovascular diseases (CVDs). According to some studies, the consumption of oily fish leads to increased levels of omega-3 PUFAs and thereafter a favourable cardiovascular prognosis; this statement was supported with epidemiological data evaluated by meta-analyses and it has been linked to higher levels of eicosapentaenoic acid (EPA) and docosahexaenoic acid (DHA).

Clinically, men who consume oily fish at least once a week had a 50 percent lower incidence of coronary heart disease (CHD) and sudden cardiac death (SCD). Mechanistically, though, it is not clear how omega-3 PUFAs work. We do not know whether it is the omega-3 PUFAs themselves that deliver this result or if it is some other fish micro-constituents of polar nature [1].

Not only that, but there is growing evidence that omega-3 PUFAs supplementation may not work in relation to CVDs. In detail, the (possible) association of omega-3 PUFAs and CVDs has been revised recently by evaluating all randomized trials on the supplementation of omega-3 PUFAs to adults; the results of 20 studies on 68,680 patients were evaluated and omega-3 PUFAs were not found to be statistically significantly associated with CVDs in various patient populations [2]. This work has ignited considerable discussion on the (possible) effect of EPA and DHA's supplementation to CVDs. Once the (supplemented) ethyl esters of EPA and DHA reach our stomach, do they undergo acid hydrolysis and oxidation? Our view is this: omega-3PUFAs, most probably, might not be able to reach the tissue target or enter blood circulation in their active form and further clinical evidence is needed on whether ethyl esters or in fact polar derivatives of omega-3 PUFAs can have an impact on CVDs.

In addition to the work of Rizos et al. [2], in 2014, another two extensive reviews have been published on the (possible) effects of omega-3 PUFAs supplementation.

In the first one, the authors have searched five electronic databases (i.e. MEDLINE, EMBASE, CENTRAL, Scopus and the International Clinical Trials Registry Platform) from inception to 6th December 2013 to identify randomized trials of omeaga-3 PUFAs supplementation (from fish or plant oils) that lasted more than 12 weeks in adults with peripheral arterial disease. Five trials enrolling 396 individuals have been included and the authors have concluded that "insufficient evidence exists to suggest a beneficial effect of omega-3 PUFAs supplementation in adults with peripheral arterial disease with regard to cardiovascular events and other serious clinical outcomes" [3].

In the second one, the authors have performed electronic searches in Pubmed, EmBase and the Cochrane Library to identify randomized controlled trials on cancer incidence, nonvascular death and total mortality. They have used relative risk (RR) to measure the effect of omega-3 PUFAs supplementation on the risk of cancer incidence, nonvascular death and total mortality using a random-effect model. They have concluded that "omega-3

PUFAs supplementation does not have an effect on cancer incidence, nonvascular death or total mortality" [4].

In the previous chapter, a detailed description on how Omacor® has been created is given. Omacor®, which is concentrated and highly purified fish oil, is also traded in the US under the name Lovaza® and it is an approved drug, by the US Food and Drug Administration, drug for treating hyperlipidemia [5].

However, the consumption of dietary marine oils may have adverse consequences. In clinical studies of Lovaza®, increased serum aspartate aminotransferase and alanine aminotransferase have been reported. These increased enzymatic activities could be evidence of liver toxicity [6].

Another postmarketing adverse reaction observed with Lovaza® is hemorrhagic diathesis [6]. Some evidence of increased risk for prostate cancer among men with high blood levels of omega-3 PUFAs has also been reported recently [7, 8].

In a recent study on the effect of Lovaza® and krill oil using mice, Spindler et al. have assessed the effect of these mixtures on the life span and mortality related pathologies of long-lived, male, B6C3F1 mice. Krill oil and Lovaza® have been administered isocalorically to mice. Krill oil was 3% and Lovaza® 11% of the oil in the diet of the mice; that in this study was the chemically defined American Institute of Nutrition (AIN)-93 M diet. The authors have analyzed serum from treated mice and have found that Lovaza® slightly increased blood urea nitrogen whereas krill oil modestly increased the levels of bilirubin, triglycerides and blood glucose. They have concluded that doses of either krill oil or Lovaza®, consistent with those recommended for human use, have decreased the life span of healthy mice. The consumption of marine oil has increased deaths associated with hemorrhagic diathesis and specific types of tumors [9].

Polar Lipids of Fish with Anti-Inflammatory Properties

Over the past decade, we have carried out research on the nutritional value of fish and we particularly focused on the lipid fractions of fish that can inhibit the aggregation of platelets and can thus have a cardioprotective effect [10, 11]. In a considerable number of fish species, the compounds that inhibit the PAF-initiated platelet aggregation have been found to belong to the class of polar lipids (PL) (see also chapter 5).

Simultaneously, we have focused on the by-products of olive industry: olive pomace (OP) is one of two major by-products of the olive oil extraction industry when using the three-phase centrifugal technology and there is the tendency of using it in several agricultural and aquacultural applications with promising results. One of the most promising applications would be to valorize it as animal and feed ingredient [12].

In order to assess this possible valorization of OP, gilthead sea bream (*Sparus aurata*) and sea bass (*Dicentrarchus labrax*) were fed with two experimental diets (8 % OP in *S. aurata* diet and 4 % OP in *D. labrax* diet), in order to examine whether enrichment of fish diet with OP would have any influence on growth performance, fatty acid composition and cardio protective properties of fish.

It has been shown that the incorporation of 8 % of OP in the fish feed has not affected the satisfactory growth in gilthead sea bream at the end of the on-growing period (90 days). The biological activity of TL obtained from gilthead sea bream fed with the OP diet was significantly increased in comparison with the gilthead sea bream fed with the fish oil (FO) diet [13].

The strong cardioprotective properties of fish fed with OP are most probably due to the fact that OP contains anti-PAF lipid components [14]. These PL of OP can enrich fish flesh when aquacultured fish are fed with OP. This use of OP in aquaculture would lead to a novel functional food by exploiting a by-product of olive industry [15].

The question though that still remains unanswered is: which specific compounds in fish or marine oils inhibit the aggregation of platelets and therefore the onset of atherosclerosis?

In order to answer this question, we have been trying to isolate the most biologically active PL fractions of fish fed with OP. The most biologically active fractions were further studied by mass spectrometry techniques such as ESMS/MS and GC–MS. Glycerophospholipid species were identified from the major classes such as phosphatidylcholine (PC), phosphatidylethanolamine (PE), phosphatidylserine (PS), phosphatidylinositol (PI), phosphatidylglycerol (PG) and phosphatidic acid (PA) containing 18:0/18:1 and 20:2/22:6 at the sn-1 and sn-2 positions respectively.

This work is the first study elucidating the structure of fish muscle PL that has been fed with OP-diet [16] and it could be thus suggested that omega-3 PUFAs are actually bioactive against CVDs when they are conjugated to a polar head, not as free acids or ethyl esters.

Therefore, OP inclusion in fish feed and the usage of this feed to produce aquacultured gilthead sea bream or sea bass has a dual beneficial impact.

Firstly, OP enriches both fish feed and fish in PL with cardioprotective properties and secondly, OP is valorized as a potential partial replacement of FO in the quest for sustainable production of fish feeds [1].

What Next? Let's Imagine…

There is considerable doubt today about whether lowering blood cholesterol is a true prerequisite in order to protect ourselves from CVDs. In fact, cholesterol can be correlated with CVDs but without being a causal factor for it. Therefore, people with high levels of High Density Lipoproteins (HDL) face no higher risk of CVDs as the ratio (and not only the absolute levels!) of LDL to HDL is also important in disease prognosis.

Taking all of the above into consideration, it is rather surprising to see that most of the studies in aquaculture do not address the nutritional value of the final produce from the consumer's point of view. People eat fish because they have been told that "fish is good for you" and this is valid and true. On top of that, aquaculture fish is even better since all raw ingredients and fish are constantly scrutinized under strict quality assurance procedures following all relevant requirements (for example, those of ISO22000, ISO9001, IFS, BRC, etc). The final product is thus fully checked in terms of safety and quality but also in terms of sensory properties.

It should be questioned: is it properly evaluated for its nutritional value against CVDs? If not, future research into the identification of fish lipids with specific cardioprotective activities could bring added value to aquaculture and be a viable marketing tool in promoting (functional) aquafeeds and fish. The commercial future could be bright if the functional properties of fish were to be emphasized on the label, after having carried out relevant bioassays. In doing so, it would be vital to assess the full lipidomic spectrum for cardioprotective activities and not only the levels of omega-3 PUFAs. Fish do contain polar lipids with strong anti-atherogenic properties [11, 16] and these molecules can be further exploited, both academically and commercially.

Let's now imagine an aquafeed company that had merged with an aquaculture company and after this merger, the resulting company merged with a snack manufacturer and then with a delicatessen high street shop. A scenario of totality. Impossible you might think. But, impossible is nothing.

Now, this total chain company uses functional aquafeeds as raw ingredients and the bioactive ingredients of the feeds pass all the way to the fish strips with olive oil and lemon that are extruded and packed in a 70g little sachet to be sold as a delicious and nutritious snack (a healthier alternative to crisps!). So, this company would trade now snacks labelled as "fish with olive oil and lemon: the Med diet in a sachet". Would you buy it? Would you consider it as an alternative and much more nutritional snack for your lunch break?

The totality described in the previous two paragraphs does not exist. However, this could/should be the driving force in aquaculture, food, nutraceutical and pharmaceutical industries today; how we can better manufacture (i.e. more cost effective, more nutritional, more "appealing") aquafeeds, with improved flavor and color, in order to produce fish and fish products with higher added value.

Fish snacks do exist in Japan (albeit not in the form described here) but not in Europe or US. So, what is missing in Europe or US in order to produce such a functional novel food? At the end of the day, Europeans and Americans are supposedly interested in following a healthy diet and are thus prepared to spend a little more money to purchase more nutritional food. Will the involved industries identify these consumer trends and become more "holistic" in their approach?

The cutting edge products that are badly needed today at the consumer level, i.e. on the super market shelf, are functional foods (or nutraceuticals derived from these functional foods) containing whole fish (not only omega-3 PUFAs!) as there is growing scientific evidence that total fish is beneficial against CVDs as opposed to omega-3 PUFAs supplements. This scientific evidence needs, thus, to be translated and transcripted by the industry into novel functional food (e.g. fish snacks) with a flavor and nutritional value better than omega-3 pills. Impossible is nothing!

REFERENCES

[1] I. Zabetakis, *J. Food Sci.* 78, R1101 (2013).

[2] E. C. Rizos, E. E. Ntzani, E. Bika, M. S. Kostapanos, and M. S. Elisaf, *JAMA* 308, 1024 (2012).

[3] J. E. Enns, A. Yeganeh, R. Zarychanski, A. M. Abou-Setta, C. Friesen, P. Zahradka, and C. G. Taylor, *BMC Cardiovascular Disorders* 14, 70 (2014).

[4] Y. F. Zhang, H. F. Gao, A. J. Hou.

[5] S. Kar, *Am. J. Ther.* 21, 56 (2011).

[6] GlaxoSmithKline, GSK medical professional information: adverse reactions, https://www.gsksource.com/gskprm/en/US/adirect/gskprm?cmd=ProductDetailPageandproduct_id=1336506912652andfeatureKey=603462#section-34084-4.

[7] J. K. Bassett, G. Severi, A. M. Hodge, R. J. Macinnis, R. A. Gibson, J. L. Hopper, D. R. English, and G. G. Giles, *Int. J. Cancer* 133, 188291 (2013).

[8] T. M. Brasky, A. K. Darke, X. Song, C. M. Tangen, P. J. Goodman, I. M. Thompson, F. L. Meyskens Jr, G. E. Goodman, L. M. Minasian, H. L. Parnes, E. A. Klein, and A. R. Kristal, *J. Natl. Cancer Inst.* 105, 1132 (2013).

[9] S. R. Spindler, P. L. Mote and J. M. Flegal, *Age* 36, 1345 (2014).

[10] T. Nomikos, H. C. Karantonis, C. Skarvelis, C. A. Demopoulos, and I. Zabetakis, *Food Chem.* 96, 29 (2006).

[11] C. Nasopoulou, A. B. Tsoupras, H. C. Karantonis, C. A. Demopoulos, and I. Zabetakis, *Lipids Health Dis.*10, 213 (2011).

[12] C. Nasopoulou and I. Zabetakis, *J. Agric. Sci.* 5, 116 (2013).

[13] C. Nasopoulou, G. Stamatakis, I. Zabetakis, and C. A. Demopoulos, *Food Chem.* 129, 1108 (2011).

[14] N. Tsantila, H. C. Karantonis, D. N. Perrea, S. E. Theocharis, D. G. Iliopoulos, S. Antonopoulou, and C. A. Demopoulos, *Mediators Inflamm.* 2007, 36204 (2007).

[15] Patent on "Production method of fish feed enriched with polar lipids and method to enrich farmed fishes" Application Number WO2014IB58759 20140203, http://worldwide.espacenet.com/publicationDetails/biblio?FT=Danddate=20140814andDB=andlocale=en_EPandCC=WOandNR=2014122571A1andKC=A1andND=1.

[16] C. Nasopoulou, T. Smith, M. Detopoulou, C. Tsikrika, L. Papaharisis, D. Barkas, and I. Zabetakis, *Food Chem.* 145, 1097 (2014).

About the Authors

Anthony P. Bimbo
Technical Consultant
International Fisheries Technology
Post Office Box 1606, 55 Cedar Lane
Kilmarnock, Virginia USA 22482-1606
Tel 804-435-3915
E-Mail apbimbo@verizon.net

I am a technical consultant with 52.5 years' experience working in the global commercial fishing industry. The first 33 years were spent with the largest fishmeal and oil producer in the USA, with 6 years directing operations, marketing and research activities for their marine oil refinery. I was the technical director on their menhaden surimi project and was co-chairman of the US Special Menhaden Task Force that submitted the Generally Recognized as Safe (GRAS) menhaden oil petition to the US FDA. I also chaired the Scientific Committee of the International Fishmeal and Fish Oil Organization (IFFO) for 7 years.

I have been consulting for 19.5 years. My projects have generally fit into 3 categories: Regulatory/Legal, Marketing and Processing. My 52+ years of experience is rather focused and unique. I have served on 9 Expert GRAS Panels for various marine oil products. I have consulted with a number of nutritional oil, pharmaceutical and food companies and assisted them in sourcing marine oils. I have also worked with the UN FAO, USAID, the US EPA and several NGO's in Alaska, the Maldive Islands, Peru, Chile and elsewhere on projects related to by-product recovery, pollution prevention and yield enhancement in the seafood industry. I've been a technical advisor to GOED (Global Organization for EPA and DHA Omega 3s) since 2007 and received their lifetime achievement award for excellence in 2009. I have worked with several microalgae companies during their initial start-up and feasibility projects. I have also been involved as an expert on several patent infringement cases.

Jana Pickova

I am professor in Food science at the Department of Food Science at the Swedish University of Agricultural Sciences (SLU). I have studied biology and chemistry and have a phd degree from 1998 in food science/chemistry.

Since 2008 I am professor at the SLU and work with fish quality and lipid composition, oxidation and health effects. I also have interest in fish nutrition and novel sources of LCPUFA for aquaculture feeds. I have intense collaboration especially with the Norwegian and Czech universities.

http://www.slu.se/en/departments/food-science/

Margaret Crumlish

Dr. Mags Crumlish is a senior lecturer at the Institute of Aquaculture, Stirling University, Scotland. She contributes towards teaching on undergraduate and postgraduate courses at Stirling and supervises several PhD students from all over the world. As an aquatic microbiologist her research focuses on the identification and characterization of bacterial pathogens affecting farmed aquatic animals, globally. She also investigates the microbial food safety of the farmed fish products sold on the international market. Her work contributes towards the sustainable production of the aquaculture sector and the safety of the aquatic seafood we consume.

margaret.crumlish@stir.ac.uk

Ioannis Zabetakis

Yannis (Ioannis) Zabetakis studied for his BSc in Chemistry in the Univ. of Athens and then spent 8 years in UK where he studied for a PhD in Food Science in the Univ. of Leeds. He did postdoctoral research on alkaloids in the Univ. of Durham and worked as a Lecturer in Food Chemistry in the Univ. of Leeds. During his lectureship in Leeds (1998-2001), he also studied for a M.Ed. in Food Chemistry.

Since 2003, he has been working in the laboratory of Food Chemistry in the Univ. of Athens (2003-2008 Lecturer of Food Chemistry, 2008-2012 tenure-track Assistant Professor of Food Chemistry and since 2012 as a Tenured Assistant Professor of Food Chemistry).

He uses e-learning as a tool for professional development in the Food Industry where he is also involved in consulting and auditing (as a Lead Auditor, HACCP/ISO). He advocates the dissemination of food science and nutrition to the public (through written articles on nutrition and food safety issues in specialised food sector magazines / newspapers and radio / tv appearances).

http://www.chem.uoa.gr/personel/Laboratories/FoodChem/cvs/zabetakis.htm

Constantina Nasopoulou

Dr. Constantina Nasopoulou is a Lecturer in Food Science and Technology at the Department of Food Science and Nutrition (D.F.S.N.) of the University of the Aegean, Greece and Co-author - Tutor of seven web-based modules of distance learning (e-learning) in Food Chemistry, Food Biotechnology and Functional Foods at the National and Kapodistrian University of Athens, Greece. Her research interests include: a) isolation and characterization of bioactive lipid micro-constituents, against atherogenesis, of either fish or olive origin, b) the impact of lipid micro-constituents on the mechanism of thrombosis, atherogenesis and hypertension and c) the formulation and production of sustainable aquacultural and agricultural feeds in order to produce functional foods with reinforced cardioprotective properties. She is a member of the Editorial Board of seven peer-reviewed international journals and Guest Editor of the special issue: "Marine Functional Food Products – Cardiovascular Diseases" of the peer-reviewed international journal "Marine Drugs". She has published 21 papers in peer-reviewed international journals, co-autthored several book chapters and edited a food tchnology textbook.

knasopoulou@aegean.webmail.gr;
cnasopoulou@chem.uoa.gr

Smaragdi Antonopoulou et al.

The team of Harokopio University consists of the following members: Dr Smaragdi Antonopoulou, Professor in Biochemistry, Director of the Laboratory "Biology, Biochemistry and Physiology", Dr Tzortzis Nomikos, Assistant Professor in Biochemistry, Dr Elisabeth Fragopoulou, Assistant Professor in Biological Chemistry, and Dr Paraskevi Detopoulou, Clinical Dietician.

The team of the Department of Nutrition and Dietetics of Harokopio University focuses on both basic and applied nutrition research. In specific, the team has an expertise a) in the isolation and characterization of micro-constituents especially of Mediterranean foods, b) in the study of basic patho-physiological mechanisms, namely inflammation, oxidative stress and thrombosis and how they are affected by food micro-constituents and c) in the metabolism and the implication of lipid mediators especially Platelet-Activating Factor (PAF) in several patho-physiological conditions. The team has published over 100 papers in peer-reviewed, leading scientific international journals, with more than 1500 citations, three invited commentary articles in International Atherosclerosis Society website, chapters in four international books and over 150 abstracts in International and Greek Conferences. The team also holds 2 patents, and has number of collaboration contracts with private bodies and SME and has also been involved as project coordinators in 17 National and European projects.

Alexis Garras et al.

Dr. Alexis Garras is a biochemist, having done his undergraduate work at Wesleyan University, Ct., USA, his MSc and PhD at the University of Bergen (1997), The Department of Medical Biochemistry, and specifically on omega-3 fatty acid biochemistry. He has worked within the field of lipidology for several pharmaceutical companies during the last 18 years, among them AstraZeneca, MSD and Boehringer Ingelheim.

Dr. David Fraser is a biochemist, with an MSc in Human Nutrition & Metabolism from Aberdeen University (1994) and a PhD in Immune & Endocrine Responses to Acute starvation, University of Oslo (2000). He has worked as a post-doc researcher on various projects in the field of immunology and diabetic microvascular complications.

Dr. Derek Tobin is a Biochemist with degrees from the Universities of Newcastle---upon---Tyne and Sheffield, UK (1993). He completed his Post-Doctoral research at the Karolinska Institute in Sweden and subsequently worked as a medical writer at GE Healthcare. He then took a position as Senior Scientist at DiaGenic ASA in Oslo.

Runar Vige is exercise physiologist by training, with an MSc degree from Norwegian School of Sport Sciences. He also holds an MBA from BI Norwegian Business School. He has worked within the field of dyslipidemia and cardiovascular disease for Pfizer and Pronova BioPharma during the last 13 years, both in clinical development roles and in cross-functional business development roles

Ida Marie Wold has an MSc degree in Chemical Engineering and Biotechnology from the Norwegian University of Science and Technology.

The authors currently work with omega-3 fatty acids at PronovaBioPharma/BASF in Oslo.

INDEX

#

A

B

C

D

E

F

G

N

O

P

Q

R

S

T

U

V

W

Y

Z